Did you know you could earn
15 AMA Category 1 CME credits
by reading this issue?

Physician Assistant Clinics subscribers can access online CME tests based on each issue to **earn up to 60 AMA Category 1 CME credits per year** (15 credits per issue, 4 issues per year).

If you are a current subscriber, visit **physicianassistant.theclinics.com/CME** to claim access and to begin taking the exams.

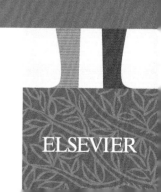

HOW IT WORKS:

- Bookmark physicianassistant.theclinics.com/CME—exams are posted online a month after each *Physician Assistant Clinics* issue publishes.

- Read the issue and pass the exam for instant AMA PRA Category 1 Credit(s)™.

- Certificates may be printed immediately upon successful completion of the exam and program evaluation.

- A personal user account (MyCME) records all exam results and credits, and allows users to save in-progress exams and complete them at a later date.

- This CME program is planned and implemented in accordance with the Essential Areas and Policies of the Accreditation Council for Continuing Medical Education through the Elsevier Office of Continuing Medical Education.

Not a subscriber to *Physician Assistant Clinics?*
Visit physicianassistant.theclinics.com
or call +1 (800) 654-2452 (USA) or +1 (314) 447-8871 (ROW)
to stay updated on the latest advancements in medicine
and earn the CME credits you need in less time!

ELSEVIER

Oncology

Editor

ALEXANDRIA GARINO

PHYSICIAN ASSISTANT CLINICS

www.physicianassistant.theclinics.com

Consulting Editor
JAMES A. VAN RHEE

July 2016 • Volume 1 • Number 3

ELSEVIER

1600 John F. Kennedy Boulevard • Suite 1800 • Philadelphia, Pennsylvania, 19103-2899

http://www.theclinics.com

PHYSICIAN ASSISTANT CLINICS Volume 1, Number 3
July 2016 ISSN 2405-7991, ISBN-13: 978-0-323-44852-9

Editor: Jessica McCool
Developmental Editor: Casey Jackson

Physician Assistant Clinics (ISSN: 2405–7991) is published quarterly by Elsevier Inc., 360 Park Avenue South, New York, NY 10010-1710. Months of issue are January, April, July, and October. Periodicals postage paid at New York, NY and additional mailing offices. Subscription prices are $150.00 per year (US individuals), $195.00 (US institutions), $100.00 (US students), $150.00 (Canadian individuals), $245.00 (Canadian institutions), $100.00 (Canadian students), $150.00 (international individuals), $245.00 (international institutions), and $100.00 (international students). Foreign air speed delivery is included in all *Clinics* subscription prices. All prices are subject to change without notice. POSTMASTER: Send address changes to *Physician Assistant Clinics*, Elsevier Periodicals Customer Service, 11830 Westline Industrial Drive, St. Louis, MO 63146. Customer Service Health Sciences Division, Subscription Customer Service, 3251 Riverport Lane, Maryland Heights, MO 63043. **Customer Service: 1-800-654-2452 (U.S. and Canada); 314-447-8871 (outside U.S. and Canada). Fax: 314-447-8029. E-mail: journalscustomerservice-usa@elsevier.com (for print support); journalsonlinesupport-usa@elsevier.com (for online support).**

Reprints. For copies of 100 or more, of articles in this publication, please contact the Commercial Reprints Department, Elsevier Inc., 360 Park Avenue South, New York, NY 10010-1710. Tel. 212-633-3874; Fax: 212-633-3820; E-mail: reprints@elsevier.com.

Physician Assistant Clinics is covered in *MEDLINE/PubMed (Index Medicus)* and *EMBASE/Excerpta Medica, Current Contents/Clinical Medicine,* and *ISI/BIOMED.*

PROGRAM OBJECTIVE

The goal of the *Physician Assistant Clinics* is to keep practicing physician assistants up to date with current clinical practice by providing timely articles reviewing the state of the art in patient care.

TARGET AUDIENCE

Physician Assistants and other healthcare professionals.

LEARNING OBJECTIVES

Upon completion of this activity, participants will be able to:
1. Review ethical considerations and improving access to cancer care.
2. Discuss symptom management in oncology, including nutrition and new pharmacological agents.
3. Recognize advances oncology treatment in such pathologies as breast cancer, ovarian cancer, and squamous cell carcinoma.

ACCREDITATION

The Elsevier Office of Continuing Medical Education (EOCME) is accredited by the Accreditation Council for Continuing Medical Education (ACCME) to provide continuing medical education for physicians.

The EOCME designates this enduring material for a maximum of 15 *AMA PRA Category 1 Credit*(s)™. Physicians should claim only the credit commensurate with the extent of their participation in the activity.

All other health care professionals requesting continuing education credit for this enduring material will be issued a certificate of participation.

DISCLOSURE OF CONFLICTS OF INTEREST

The EOCME assesses conflict of interest with its instructors, faculty, planners, and other individuals who are in a position to control the content of CME activities. All relevant conflicts of interest that are identified are thoroughly vetted by EOCME for fair balance, scientific objectivity, and patient care recommendations. EOCME is committed to providing its learners with CME activities that promote improvements or quality in healthcare and not a specific proprietary business or a commercial interest.

The planning committee, staff, authors and editors listed below have identified no financial relationships or relationships to products or devices they or their spouse/life partner have with commercial interest related to the content of this CME activity:

Christine Cambareri, PharmD, BCPS, BCOP; Carolyn M. Canonica, MMSc, PA-C; Joseph Daniel; Anjali Fortna; Jessica Gahres, PA-C, MS; Alexandria Garino, MS, PA-C; Elizabeth M. Garland, MPAS, PA-C; Heather M. Hylton, MS, PA-C, DFAAPA; Casey Jackson; Yvonne H. Jee, MS, PA-C; Katherine L. Kunstel, MMSc, PA-C; Sharyn L. Kurtz, PA-C, MPAS, MA; Jessica McCool; Katayoun Moini, MHS, PA-C, RD, CNSC; Courtney Moller, PA-C, MS; Ian Nagus, PA-C, MS; Carmen F. Nobre, PharmD, BCOP; Brittney O'Grady, MMS, PA-C; Lauren C. Parker, MPAS, PA-C, RD; Tamera Plair, MS, PA-C; Kristine Prazak, PA-C, MS; Teresa G. Scardino, MPAS, PA-C; Jerrad M. Stoddard, MA, MS, PA-C; Megan Suermann; Laura A. Tuttle, PharmD, BCOP.

The planning committee, staff, authors and editors listed below have identified financial relationships or relationships to products or devices they or their spouse/life partner have with commercial interest related to the content of this CME activity:

James A. Van Rhee, MS, PA-C, DFAAPA receives royalties/patents from Kaplan, Inc.

UNAPPROVED/OFF-LABEL USE DISCLOSURE

The EOCME requires CME faculty to disclose to the participants:
1. When products or procedures being discussed are off-label, unlabelled, experimental, and/or investigational (not US Food and Drug Administration [FDA] approved); and
2. Any limitations on the information presented, such as data that are preliminary or that represent ongoing research, interim analyses, and/or unsupported opinions. Faculty may discuss information about pharmaceutical agents that is outside of FDA-approved labelling. This information is intended solely for CME and is not intended to promote off-label use of these medications. If you have any questions, contact the medical affairs department of the manufacturer for the most recent prescribing information.

TO ENROLL

The CME program is available to all *Physician Assistant Clinics* subscribers at no additional fee. To subscribe to the *Physician Assistant Clinics*, call customer service at 1-800-654-2452 or sign up online at www.physicianassistant.theclinics.com.

METHOD OF PARTICIPATION

In order to claim credit, participants must complete the following:

1. Complete enrolment as indicated above.
2. Read the activity.
3. Complete the CME Test and Evaluation. Participants must achieve a score of 70% on the test. All CME Tests and Evaluations must be completed online.

CME INQUIRIES/SPECIAL NEEDS

For all CME inquiries or special needs, please contact elsevierCME@elsevier.com.

Contributors

CONSULTING EDITOR

JAMES A. VAN RHEE, MS, PA-C, DFAAPA
Associate Professor, Program Director, Yale University, Yale Physician Associate
Program, New Haven, Connecticut

EDITOR

ALEXANDRIA GARINO, MS, PA-C
Assistant Professor, Yale School of Medicine, Physician Associate Program; Physician
Assistant, Malignant Hematology, Yale Cancer Center, New Haven, Connecticut

AUTHORS

CHRISTINE CAMBARERI, PharmD, BCPS, BCOP
Perelman Center for Advanced Medicine, Abramson Cancer Center, Hospital of the
University of Pennsylvania, Philadelphia, Pennsylvania

CAROLYN M. CANONICA, MMSc, PA-C
Physician Assistant, Adult Bone Marrow Transplant Service, Department of Medicine,
Memorial Sloan Kettering Cancer Center, New York, New York

JESSICA GAHRES, PA-C, MS
Department of Medicine, Gynecologic Medical Oncology, Memorial Sloan Kettering
Cancer Center, New York, New York

ELIZABETH M. GARLAND, MPAS, PA-C
Physician Assistant, Department of Head and Neck Surgery, University of Texas MD
Anderson Cancer Center, Houston, Texas

HEATHER M. HYLTON, MS, PA-C, DFAAPA
Lead Physician Assistant, Memorial Sloan Kettering Cancer Center (MSKCC), Department
of Medicine, New York, New York

YVONNE H. JEE, MS, PA-C
Department of Stem Cell Transplantation and Cellular Therapy, The University of Texas
MD Anderson Cancer Center, Houston, Texas

KATHERINE L. KUNSTEL, MMSc, PA-C
Assistant Clinical Professor; Director of Admissions, Department of Physician Assistant
Studies, College of Health Professions, Pace University-Lenox Hill Hospital, New York,
New York; Inpatient Oncology Physician Assistant, Smilow Cancer Hospital at Yale-New
Haven Hospital, New Haven, Connecticut; Inpatient Bone Marrow Transplant and
Malignant Hematology Physician Assistant, New York-Presbyterian Hospital, New York,
New York

SHARYN L. KURTZ, PA-C, MPAS, MA
Lymphoma Service, Department of Medicine, Physician Assistant Clinics on Oncology, Memorial Sloan Kettering Cancer Center, New York, New York

KATAYOUN MOINI, MHS, PA-C, RD, CNSC
PA Program Director; Assistant Professor, Charles R. Drew University of Medicine and Science, Los Angeles, California

COURTNEY MOLLER, PA-C, MS
Dana Farber Cancer Institute, Boston, Massachusetts

IAN NAGUS, PA-C, MS
Mass General/North Shore Cancer Center, Danvers, Massachusetts

CARMEN F. NOBRE, PharmD, BCOP
Department of Pharmacy, Smilow Cancer Hospital at Yale New Haven, New Haven, Connecticut

BRITTNEY O'GRADY, MMS, PA-C
MD Anderson Cancer Center, Department of Plastic Surgery, Houston, Texas

LAUREN C. PARKER, MPAS, PA-C, RD
Physician Assistant, Department of Head and Neck Surgery, University of Texas MD Anderson Cancer Center, Houston, Texas

TAMERA PLAIR, MS, PA-C
Department of Stem Cell Transplantation and Cellular Therapy, The University of Texas MD Anderson Cancer Center, Houston, Texas

KRISTINE PRAZAK, PA-C, MS
Assistant Professor, Department of Physician Assistant Studies, New York Institute of Technology, Old Westbury, New York

TERESA G. SCARDINO, MPAS, PA-C
Memorial Sloan Kettering Cancer Center (MSKCC), Lymphoma Service, New York, New York

JERRAD M. STODDARD, MA, MS, PA-C
Department of Stem Cell Transplantation and Cellular Therapy, The University of Texas MD Anderson Cancer Center, Houston, Texas

LAURA A. TUTTLE, PharmD, BCOP
Department of Pharmacy, Smilow Cancer Hospital at Yale New Haven, New Haven, Connecticut

Contents

Nutrition in Cancer Care   363

Katayoun Moini

> Cancer and the treatment of cancer can impact the nutritional status of our patients. Medical providers can significantly improve the quality of life for patients with cancer by intervening early and often, building rapport, and implementing a daily process for individualizing nutrition support. This article focuses on unpleasant nutrition-related effects of cancer and cancer treatments and provides strategies to improve the nutrition status of patients. It is up to medical providers to emphasize the importance of nutrition in our patients and demand these issues be addressed early through patient education and expert consultation.

Oncology: Symptom Management   375

Ian Nagus and Courtney Moller

> This article presents the concept of palliative care, describes the principles of symptom management, and provides examples of potential treatment options for these common complaints specific to patients living with a cancer diagnosis.

Oncologic Emergencies   397

Katherine L. Kunstel

> Patients with cancer and those undergoing treatment for cancer are at risk for potentially life-threatening complications, which are collectively termed, *oncologic emergencies*. Many of these patients present to the emergency room or to their primary care provider when they become ill, so recognition of these conditions and proper intervention is essential for oncology clinicians and those who practice outside of oncology. Common oncologic emergencies include febrile neutropenia, hypercalcemia of malignancy, and tumor lysis syndrome. Knowledge of the risk factors, pathophysiology, presenting features, diagnostic workup, and appropriate intervention is essential to provide the best care for these patients.

Ovarian cancer is the most deadly gynecologic malignancy. It continues to be elusive to diagnosis because its initial presentation can mimic common medical conditions. Primary care clinicians, and those working in women's health, need to be aware of the subtle signs associated with ovarian cancer. Identifying these early on can improve outcomes; early diagnosis and treatment leads to greater survival rates. There continues to be efforts to improved treatment. However, currently there is no effective screening method to detect early stage disease. This article aims to educate the clinician about symptoms, appropriate workup, referral, diagnosis, and treatment of ovarian cancer.

With the ever-increasing complexity of health care delivery, this article demonstrates how the development of a Physician/Physician Assistant (MD/PA) team can positively impact health care delivery. With an increase in demand for oncology services anticipated in the future, coupled with an anticipated shortage of clinicians to provide these services, increasing access and productivity are paramount. This article discusses how PA-lead initiatives were implemented in an outpatient lymphoma service and how the evolution of independent PA clinics has been able to positively impact the way care is delivered across multiple domains of the cancer continuum and improve access for patients.

The aim of the present study is to provide a brief review of prosthesis-based and autologous-based breast reconstruction. The study focuses on the timeline behind reconstruction, the effect of radiation, and the manner in which the appropriate surgical method is based. Regarding autologous reconstruction, the review provides a brief summary behind the factors optimizing success as well as the role of the physician assistant in flap-based reconstruction.

Ethical considerations are an important aspect of a physician assistant's clinical work in oncology. Separate from legal implications, ethical deliberation involves considering the best moral course of action for a patient, with the goal of providing optimal interdisciplinary care. This article investigates key ethical issues pertaining to physician assistant care of the oncology patient.

Oncology
PHYSICIAN ASSISTANT CLINICS

RELATED INTEREST

Clinics in Geriatric Medicine, February 2016 (Vol. 32, Issue 1)
Geriatric Oncology
Harvey Jay Cohen and Arati V. Rao, *Editors*
Available at: http://www.geriatric.theclinics.com/

THE CLINICS ARE AVAILABLE ONLINE!
Access your subscription at:
www.theclinics.com

Dedication

In Loving Memory of Yvonne Hsu Jee

 CrossMark

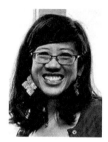

Yvonne Hsu Jee

Yvonne Hsu Jee started her career as a Physician Assistant in Stem Cell Transplant at MD Anderson Cancer Center upon graduating from Baylor College of Medicine in 2000. During her 16-year tenure, she made a profound impact on numerous colleagues and patients and was an asset to the department and institution. She served as the PA supervisor, facilitated bone marrow donor drives for the National Marrow Donor Program, participated in various organizational committees, and most recently, coauthored a review article in this issue of *Physician Assistant Clinics*.

In addition to excelling in her clinical duties, Yvonne was devoted to her church and community. She held Bible studies for local colleges, embarked on several mission trips to China, and loved venturous sports, including skiing and snowboarding. Crafts were her niche, and she did everything with originality. The latter part of her life was the most meaningful for her. She married the love of her life in January 2015 and welcomed a precious baby boy, Jonah, on December 21, 2015. Although Yvonne's life was short-lived, she leaves a lasting legacy through her numerous accomplishments. She is remembered well by her family, friends, colleagues, and patients.

Physician Assist Clin 1 (2016) xi
http://dx.doi.org/10.1016/j.cpha.2016.04.002
2405-7991/16/$ – see front matter © 2016 Published by Elsevier Inc.

physicianassistant.theclinics.com

Foreword

Oncology

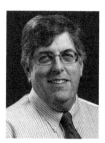

James A. Van Rhee, MS, PA-C, DFAAPA
Consulting Editor

This issue of *Physician Assistant Clinics* is of special interest to me. For years I worked in oncology before moving full time into academics. During those years, I developed a number of special relationships with the patients and their families, learned to deal with issues related to death and dying, and developed a sense of the whole patient not just a disease. This issue in Oncology covers many medical topics, but also discusses transplantation, symptom management specific to the oncology patient, and ethics in oncology.

A recent report by the American Society of Clinical Oncologists[1] predicts a significant shortage of oncology providers by 2020. While 54% of oncologists already work with physician assistants and nurse practitioners, more are needed. One option the study proposed was the increased use of physician assistants and nurse practitioners. In 2010, Ross and colleagues[2] studied the role of physician assistants in oncology and noted that many assumed high-level responsibilities that are a positive asset to the health care team in the care of oncology patients.

Fellow Yale School of Medicine colleague, Alexandria Garino, MS, PA-C, Assistant Professor at the Yale Physician Associate Program, is the guest editor for this issue, and she has selected a wide variety of topics and excellent authors from some of the leading oncology centers in the country. In this issue, we have articles for the oncology physician assistant and physician assistants in primary care. For the oncology physician assistant, Cambareri, Nobre, and Tuttle provide an in-depth discussion of new pharmaceutical agents used in oncology with a focus on targeted therapy such as monoclonal antibodies and immunomodulatory agents. For those of you interested in improving access to care, the article by Hylton and Scardino discusses the development of the MD/PA team on a lymphoma service. Stoddard, Plair, and Jee discuss the management of graft-versus-host diseases, and Prazak and Gahres provide a review of recent advances in ovarian cancer.

There is also a fine selection of articles for those working in primary care that see oncology patients, which I would imagine is just about everyone. Kunstel describes

Physician Assist Clin 1 (2016) xiii–xiv
http://dx.doi.org/10.1016/j.cpha.2016.04.003
2405-7991/16/$ – see front matter © 2016 Published by Elsevier Inc.

physicianassistant.theclinics.com

the presentation, evaluation, and treatment of some common oncologic emergencies. Nagus and Moller provide a review of the management of various symptoms seen in the oncology patient. Garland and Parker provide a review of human papillomavirus–associated oropharyngeal carcinoma, and Moini provides an excellent review of nutrition in the cancer patient.

Of special interest to me is the article by Kurtz, who discusses the ethical considerations in oncology. I think you will find this article interesting and thought provoking.

I hope you enjoy the third issue of *Physician Assistant Clinics*. Our next issue will provide you with a review of the latest in Pediatrics.

James A. Van Rhee, MS, PA-C, DFAAPA
Yale University
Yale Physician Associate Program
100 Church Street South, Suite A250
New Haven, CT 06519, USA

E-mail address:
james.vanrhee@yale.edu

REFERENCES

1. Erikson C, Salsberg E, Forte G, et al. Future supply and demand for oncologists: challenges to assuring access to oncology services. J Oncol Pract 2007;3(2): 79–86.
2. Ross AC, Polansky MN, Parker PA, et al. Understanding the role of physician assistants in oncology. J Oncol Pract 2010;6(1):26–30.

Preface

Wanted: More Oncology Physician Assistants

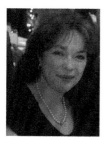

Alexandria Garino, MS, PA-C
Editor

Care of the patient with cancer is more hopeful—and more complex—today than ever before. Because of advancements in prevention, early detection, treatment, and supportive care, patients are living longer and with better quality of life. Advances are emerging at a rapid rate, fueled in part by our understanding of tumor biology and the human genome. Diseases such as renal cell carcinoma, melanoma, and non–small cell lung cancer, once limited to surgical resection and radiation, are now being treated with novel therapies that cleverly exploit new molecular pathways. In 2015 alone, the US Food and Drug Administration approved 10 new cancer treatments. Similarly, surgical and radiology techniques continue to become more sophisticated and refined.[1] The outcome of this momentum is obvious. The American Cancer Society estimated that in January 2014 there were approximately 14.5 million cancer survivors. That is a remarkable increase from the estimated 3 million survivors in 1971, when President Richard Nixon signed into law the National Cancer Act and launched the war on cancer.[2]

Physician assistants (PAs), along with our nursing colleagues, are at the front lines of the war on cancer and provide competent, compassionate, and cost-effective care.[3] Oncology PAs work wherever patients with cancer are found, yet we make up only a small percentage of the PA workforce. According to some estimates, less than 3% of practicing PAs work in oncology.[4] Our broad education, inherent team focus, and experience with delegated autonomy make us natural members of the multidimensional team needed to care for today's complex patients. Cancer care needs more PAs. PAs who work in this specialty know that we have some of the greatest PA jobs in the world. Not only are our clinical days rich and filled with varied responsibilities but also we develop close, significant clinical relationships with our patients. In short, our work is meaningful and satisfying.

The current issue of *Physician Assistant Clinics* is a celebration of these dedicated clinicians and of the patients who inspire us. To that end, articles in this Oncology issue

Physician Assist Clin 1 (2016) xv–xvi
http://dx.doi.org/10.1016/j.cpha.2016.04.001
2405-7991/16/$ – see front matter © 2016 Elsevier Inc. All rights reserved.
physicianassistant.theclinics.com

were curated with three goals in mind. First, cancer care has become technologically and scientifically intricate and requires the PA to keep abreast of latest advances. Therefore, the issue provides updates for the PA already working in oncology and provides insight into other disease states perhaps not encountered in our daily practice. In addition, topics such as ethics in oncology care and best practice guidelines for the MD/PA patient-centered team are explored.

Second, the issue strives to make the intricacies of cancer care more obvious to the general practice clinician. Team-based care of the patient with cancer involves many individuals, including the primary care team. Nononcology clinicians often encounter our active-treatment patients and cancer survivors. Therefore, articles are offered with the general practitioner in mind so that they might better understand what contributes to certain clinical presentations and what explains risk profiles particular to our unique patient population.

Third, the issue attempts to showcase the good work done by experienced oncology PAs around the country. I direct the reader's attention to the issue's table of contents. Authors from some of the country's preeminent academic cancer centers have contributed work to this issue. Also, the reader will notice that, with the exception of several of our valued oncology pharmacist colleagues, all articles are written by PAs.

Enjoy this installment of *Physician Assistant Clinics* Oncology.

Alexandria Garino, MS, PA-C
Yale School of Medicine
Physician Associate Program
100 Church Street South, Suite A250
New Haven, CT 06519, USA

E-mail address:
alexandria.garino@yale.edu

REFERENCES

1. American Society of Clinical Oncology Clinical Cancer Advances 2016. Available at: http://www.cancerprogress.net/sites/cancerprogress.net/files/asco-cca16-web-updated.pdf.
2. American Cancer Society. Cancer Treatment & Survivorship Facts & Figures 2014-2015. Available at: http://www.cancer.org/acs/groups/content/@research/documents/document/acspc-042801.pdf.
3. Kosty MP, Acheson AK, Tetzlaff ED. Clinical oncology practice 2015: preparing for the future. American Society of Clinical Oncology Education Book 2015;E622–7. http://dx.doi.org/10.14694/EdBook_AM.2015.35.e622.
4. Ross AC, Polansky MN, Parker PA, et al. Understanding the role of physician assistants in oncology. J Oncol Pract 2010;6(1):26–30.

Nutrition in Cancer Care

Katayoun Moini, MHS, PA-C, RD, CNSC

KEYWORDS

- Nutrition • Cancer • Treatment

KEY POINTS

- Specialized medical nutrition therapy is a crucial component of medical management in the oncology patient.
- Early identification of nutrition related side effects during cancer treatment is an essential component of tailored and individualized medical nutrition therapy.
- Early and ongoing nutrition assessment is necessary to identify macro and micronutrient needs.

Let food be thy medicine and medicine be thy food

—Hippocrates

INTRODUCTION

Food: We all need it, crave it, and rarely go a day without it. So why do we allow patients with life-altering disease processes, undergoing invasive therapies, go days, weeks, and even months without adequate nourishment? Would a coach allow an elite athlete to perform even one day without proper nourishment? Would a parent allow a child to not eat for days? Would you be okay with a job that did not allow you to eat during work hours? Instead of using common sense, we turn to studies to validate whether or not it is acceptable for our patients to not receive nourishment.

The importance of individualized nutrition support for patients with cancer cannot be overemphasized. Good nutrition is necessary for our patients to achieve positive outcomes and improved quality of life.

Burning More and Eating Less

Both cancer and cancer treatment negatively influence patients' nutrition status. Malnutrition caused by weight loss, anorexia, and gastrointestinal abnormalities results in inadequate nutrient intake and impaired nutrient absorption. The phenomenon known as cancer cachexia (CC) is characterized by anorexia, involuntary weight loss, progressive wasting of lean body mass and adipose tissue, and hypermetabolism.[1–4]

Disclosures: None.
Charles R. Drew University of Medicine & Science, Los Angeles, CA, USA
E-mail address: Katayounmoini@cdrewu.edu

Physician Assist Clin 1 (2016) 363–374
http://dx.doi.org/10.1016/j.cpha.2016.03.001
2405-7991/16/$ – see front matter © 2016 Elsevier Inc. All rights reserved.

Tumor factors proposed to be mechanisms contributing to CC include

- Proinflammatory cytokines
- Proteolysis-inducing factors
- Lipid-mobilizing factors

Treatment of cancer involves multiple modalities all of which can further contributes to malnutrition. Radiation involving the gastrointestinal tract may cause

- Dysgeusia
- Xerostomia
- Odynophagia and dysphagia
- Diarrhea
- Malabsorption

Surgical treatment involving the gastrointestinal tract may cause

- Delayed gastric emptying
- Malabsorption
- Nutrient deficiencies
- Dumping syndrome
- Glycemic abnormalities

Cytotoxic chemotherapy, immunotherapy, and treatment with corticosteroids and sex hormone analogues can cause additional undesirable side effects:

- Fluid and electrolyte imbalance
- Glycemic abnormalities
- Nausea and vomiting
- Diarrhea
- Nitrogen loss
- Oral and intestinal mucosal inflammation and degradation

Intervene Early, Intervene Often, and, in Other Words, Do Not Get Behind the 8 Ball

Communicating and building rapport with your patients is key to this process. Educate your patients about the potential implications of malnutrition before treatment is even initiated. Provide your patients with options to start improving their nutrition status before the onset of negative symptoms, and provide education about enteral nutrition (EN) and parenteral nutrition (PN) early in the process. Advocate for your patients, and empower your patients to advocate for themselves by educating them about the positive impact of nutrition intervention early in treatment. A negative perception of nutrition intervention (for example, use of tube feeding) can significantly delay and negatively impact the initiation of much-needed nutrition support.

Nutrition Pays a Price

There are multiple cancer therapy modalities, all of which have a negative effect on normal cells, tissues, and organs. Disruption of gastrointestinal function is a common adverse effect of therapy. Additional symptoms of fatigue, dysgeusia, and anorexia further diminish pleasure associated with food or nutrition. In fact, nutrition often becomes a subject of contention and stress for patients.[5]

Assess and Reassess on a Continuum

Determining and providing adequate and appropriate nutrition support is an ongoing process. The involvement of a qualified nutrition support team is essential for successful outcomes. The nutrition support plan must be treated the same as the clinical therapeutic plan, constantly adjusted to meet daily nutritional changes. The nutrition support team should consist of an experienced certified nutrition support dietitian, pharmacist, case manager, social worker and the medical provider overseeing the patient's care. Ideally, nutrition goals for calorie, protein, micronutrients and fluids should be determined before initiation of cancer therapy and will depend upon diagnosis, specific therapies, nutrition status, prognosis, comorbidities, organ function, performance status, and individual patient beliefs and preferences. Intervention strategies will depend on measured outcomes, such as fluctuations in weight, changes in negative and positive acute phase proteins, and gastrointestinal symptoms.[6]

Nutrient requirements for calories may vary from 25 to 35 kcal/kg/d and for protein from 1.0 to 2.5 g/kg/d. Inadequate or excessive provision of either calories or protein may have detrimental physiologic consequences; however, adequate provision can improve nutrition status, response to therapy, and reduction in symptoms. Calculation of energy expenditure can be particularly challenging, as predictive equations may underestimate or overestimate requirements. Utilization of advanced assessment tools, such as indirect calorimetry and measurement of negative and positive acute phase proteins, help improve accuracy of the nutrition support prescription.[7–9]

Fluid, electrolyte, and micronutrient calculations will be influenced by gastrointestinal symptoms, medication effects, comorbidities, and intake. Daily fine-tuning may often be required.

Assessment of Nutritional Requirements and Nutrition Status

The involvement of a registered dietitian with experience in specialized nutrition support is critical for the appropriate and adequate provision of nutrients to patients undergoing cancer therapies. Specialized education and training allow for an evidence-based, aggressive approach early in the course of treatment. As mentioned previously, multiple factors occurring during cancer therapy predispose patients to malnutrition or nutritional risk, including but not limited to reduced nutrient intake, absorption, and utilization occurring simultaneously with increased nutrient losses and requirements. The process of performing a nutrition assessment is similar to performing a comprehensive history and physical examination; however, the focus is all nutrition. The process includes obtaining a nutrition assessment focused on the following:

- Diet history[10]
  - Current nutrient deficiencies or nutritional issues
  - Food aversions and preferences
  - Dietary restrictions
  - Meal and snack consumption patterns and intake
  - Intentional and unintentional weight changes
  - Bowel routine and habits
  - Level of activity
- Medical history
  - Identify acute and chronic illnesses that may influence nutrition status
  - Surgeries or procedures involving the gastrointestinal system or alimentary tract
- Social history
  - Tobacco, alcohol, and illicit drug use
  - Financial resources influencing access to nutrition and food purchasing
  - Living conditions
  - Meal planning and preparation capabilities

- ○ Religious and spiritual beliefs
- ○ Support system
- Medication history and active medications
  - ○ Review for potential drug-nutrient interactions
  - ○ Review for medication-induced nutrient deficiencies or toxicities
  - ○ Radiation therapy involving the head, neck, or gastrointestinal tract
  - ○ Chemotherapy-induced nutrient deficiencies or toxicities
  - ○ Use of vitamin, herbal, or alternative supplements
- Allergies to foods

The process continues by obtaining and evaluating anthropometric and laboratory data and finally is completed through clinical evaluation and estimation of nutritional requirements.

Anthropometric data includes body frame, height, and weight. These data are used to calculate nutritional needs based on one of the following as a point of reference:

- Ideal body weight
- Adjusted body weight
  - ○ Adjusted for obesity, paralysis, and amputations
- Actual body weight
- Usual body weight

Using the correct weight when calculating nutritional, fluid, and electrolyte requirements is vital to prevent complications of underfeeding or overfeeding patients. This calculation will also assist with determining the degree and severity of malnutrition.[11]

Performing a nutrition-focused physical examination may reveal additional elements that affect overall nutritional status. A systematic approach to the physical examination should be used with particular attention to nutrition-related pathologies. Assessment of *energy expenditure* is the next step in determining nutritional requirements. Energy expenditure calculation is challenging in the setting of acute illness with formulas often underestimating or overestimating energy needs. Calculation involves estimation of resting energy expenditure. The most accurate measure is through indirect calorimetry by measurement of oxygen consumption, carbon dioxide production, and minute ventilation. Limitations of this method include:

- Oxygen setting greater than 50% on ventilator
- Acceptance and utilization by hospital staff
- More time intensive than calculation methods
- Excludes insensible losses of the bowel and skin
- Measures resting energy requirements and may still require provision of a stress or activity factor if patients are ambulatory

Other methods for calculating energy expenditure include:

- Predictive equations
- Requirements based on kilocalories per kilogram of body weight (using the appropriately calculated body weight)
- Body surface area

These methods are quick and do not require specialized equipment; however, clinical judgment is required for selection of the correct weight and stress factor calculation.[12]

Assessment of protein requirements includes first determining rates of protein turn-over, synthesis, breakdown, and oxidation during times of stress. Several tools can be used to help determine the appropriate provision of protein in the nutrition prescription, including anthropometric data, gastrointestinal absorption and digestion capability, nitrogen balance studies, hepatic and renal function, and laboratory assays, such as serum transport proteins. All of these tools, however, have drawbacks and should not be solely relied on to determine nutrition status, particularly in times of stress and inflammatory metabolic processes.[11]

Assessment of lipid requirements varies depending on type of disease manifestations and degree of stress. Adequate essential fatty acid intake is necessary to prevent deficiency and related complications. Assessment of lipid metabolism, degree of stress, and appropriate type of lipid provision is another essential component of nutrition evaluation by the nutrition support team.[13]

The correct selection of appropriate macronutrients to fulfill calculated energy, protein, and lipid requirements can be determined once specific macronutrient requirements are established.

Specialized Nutrition Support

Oral intake is the first step to specialized nutrition support. Increase oral intake by implementing calorie- and protein-dense foods in small portions eaten frequently throughout the day. Incorporate liquid and solid calorie- and protein-dense supplements within this plan.

EN therapy and PN therapy are both options for patients with cancer. Both may be used alone, in conjunction, or as a supplement to oral intake. Both EN and PN have indications and contraindications, which must be investigated by the nutrition support team. Both modalities are options for aggressive nutrition support when oral intake becomes inadequate to meet nutritional goals. Discussing EN and PN early in the treatment process with patients is essential, as both modalities may be viewed as negative interventions by patients, resulting in a delay in initiation of necessary treatment. Both forms of SNS can be tailored to address specific nutritional needs and deficiencies.[14]

Help Is on the Way: Pharmacologic Options

Multiple pharmacologic agents are available to assist with symptom management and can be implemented early in the treatment plan. As with any intervention, adverse effects must first be considered before implementation. A thorough review by the nutrition support team of the patients' current condition and treatment plan will help determine the most appropriate pharmacologic intervention. Options include:

- Progestational agents: stimulate appetite and weight gain
- Glucocorticoids: reduce anorexia, nausea, and vomiting
- Cannabinoids: stimulate appetite and reduce nausea and vomiting

Often the side effect of a medication may alleviate or exacerbate additional symptoms. Diligent review of medications, side effects, and current symptoms will assist with proper pharmacologic intervention selection.[15–17] The antiemetics listed next have noted side effects that may be advantageous in certain circumstances:

- Scopolamine patch: Anticholinergic activity may help reduce diarrhea.
- Metoclopramide: Prokinetic activity may assist with delayed gastric emptying in patients experiencing fullness and early satiety.
- Serotonin antagonists: May assist with the reduction of diarrhea.[18]

Combating Symptoms with Nutrition

Many nutritional strategies can be implemented to assist with symptoms resulting from cancer treatment therapies. Even small improvements in the symptoms listed next, can have positive effects on nutrition status.

Anorexia (Poor Appetite)

Loss of appetite is a common symptom negatively affecting nutrition status. Factors contributing to loss of appetite include stress, anxiety, medication and therapy side effects, and reduced physical activity. This continued loss of appetite and interest in food often escalates to tension during mealtimes and even toward well-meaning friends and family members trying to encourage oral intake. A few strategies listed next may help improve nutrition status when appetite is poor[19,20]:

- Encourage patients to take advantage of times or days appetite improves.
- Encourage small portions of calorie- and protein-dense foods throughout the day.
- Encourage consistent grazing on dense but small snacks every 1 to 3 hours.
- Boost fluids: Although staying hydrated is important, avoid filling up on calorie-less fluids. Encourage sports drinks, fruit nectars, smoothies, and liquid supplements in small amounts throughout the day. Give soups a boost with nonfat milk powder and a small amount of grated cheese or olive and canola oil.
- Boost foods: Add nonfat milk powder to foods. Add it to milk, soup, mashed sweet or regular potatoes, muffins, puddings, eggs, pancakes, oatmeal, waffles, and pancakes.
- Snack smart: Encourage strawberry Newtons, pretzels, baked tortilla or potato chips, cinnamon graham crackers, wheat thins, animal crackers, gingersnaps, gummy candies, granola, vanilla wafers, and marshmallows. Add jelly, jam, or peanut butter to crackers and fruit.
- Boost fruit: Encourage fruit canned in light syrup, applesauce, dried fruit, banana chips, and fruit leathers.
- Boost dairy: Encourage string or mozzarella cheese, flavored yogurt, sorbet, flavored milk, and low-fat cottage cheese. Add parmesan cheese to soups and scrambled eggs.
- Boost protein: Encourage thin-sliced cooked chicken, turkey, or ham; tuna canned in water; scrambled eggs, egg beaters, or salted boiled eggs; beef or turkey jerky; and protein bars or liquid supplements containing more than 10 g of protein and less than 10 g of fat per bar.
- Encourage patients to eat what they like. Patients may not desire the healthiest options. Remember adequate consumption of calories and protein is most crucial.
- Encourage patients to eat when hungry rather than sticking to a meal schedule.
- Incorporate an appetite stimulant into the diet.
- Encourage increasing activity 1 hour before meals if possible.

Early Satiety

Patients undergoing cancer therapy will often complain of feeling full after having consumed only a small amount of food. The strategies for managing early satiety are similar to those used to manage a poor appetite. However, a few additional approaches should be used[21]:

- Limit dietary fiber to less than 3 g per serving.
- Increase protein intake to at least 15 g per meal.
- Avoid carbonated beverages and excessive beverages before meals.

Nausea and Vomiting

Nausea can dramatically decrease the amount of nutrients consumed. The following strategies may help decrease triggers of nausea while increasing the amount of nutrients consumed.

Addressing nausea early in the course of treatment, experimenting with multiple strategies, and empowering your patients to be proactive when symptoms arise are essential for successful management. Multiple pharmacologic therapies exist that successfully alleviate nausea. Incorporating medications before the onset of nausea and then treating breakthrough nausea will improve symptom relief.

Adequate intravenous or oral hydration is imperative during times of nausea.

Recognizing triggers of nausea is also an important aspect of patient education. Triggers may include certain odors, brushing teeth, and movement, such as riding in a vehicle. A bland diet with incorporation of isotonic liquids may help reduce or alleviate nausea[21]:

- Provide small, frequent meals.
- Encourage consumption of liquids between instead of with meals.
- Avoid high-fat, fried, and spicy foods.
- Encourage sipping liquids through a straw.
- Avoid foods with strong odors.
- Avoid lying down for at least 2 hours after eating.
- Prescribe an antiemetic 15 to 30 minutes before eating.

Encourage the consumption of the following foods:

- Toast and crackers
- Pretzels
- Vanilla Wafers
- Gingersnaps
- Angel food cake
- Oatmeal or cream of rice
- Baked or broiled chicken or turkey breast without skin
- Yogurt
- Sherbet
- Canned fruits
- Broth
- Popsicles

Discourage the consumption of the following foods:

- Fatty, greasy, and fried foods
- Very spicy foods
- Hot foods
- Foods with strong odors

Diarrhea

Diarrhea is a frequently encountered symptom of cancer therapy resulting from multiple causes, including treatment side effects, medications, diet, and infectious microorganisms. In addition to contributing to malnutrition, dehydration, and electrolyte imbalance, diarrhea is uncomfortable, inconvenient, and discouraging.

Determining the cause of diarrhea will guide the treatment. Some simple medication adjustments can lessen osmotic load in the gut and improve diarrhea. When using medications containing sugar alcohols, such as mannitol, sorbitol, and xylitol, dilute the medication with 20 to 30 mL of water. Many elixir-form medications contain these ingredients. Additionally, be vigilant about evaluating medications taken either orally or given enterally to treat electrolyte imbalances. Magnesium- and potassium-containing medications given orally are frequently associated with gastrointestinal upset and diarrhea, further contributing to the electrolyte imbalance. Strategies to lessen these side effects include[21]

- Diluting elixir medications with water
- Reducing dosage of oral electrolyte replacement medications when possible
- Adjusting frequency or timing of oral electrolyte replacement
- Switching to intravenous delivery of oral electrolyte replacement during times of diarrhea exacerbation
- Substituting less irritating forms of the medication, such as enteric coated medications when possible
- Using nutrition to deliver necessary electrolytes
- Monitoring laboratory values closely and being diligent about adjusting oral or intravenous electrolyte replacement based on serum electrolyte trends to avoid need for bolus dosing

The following list of low-residue foods eliminates foods that provoke diarrhea and encourages foods that are easier to digest and tolerate:

- Increase fluid intake with sports beverages, cranberry juice, diluted grape juice, rice milk, warm decaffeinated tea, broth, popsicles, flat ginger ale, coconut water.
- Reduce lactose intake: Avoid milk and encourage low-fat string cheese and low-fat yogurt without fruit.
- Avoid foods high in insoluble fiber (more than 2 g per serving): raw vegetables, raw fruit, and bread and cereal with more than 2 g of fiber per serving.
- Avoid high-fat fried or greasy foods.
- Increase high-potassium-containing foods (orange juice, bananas [raw or dried], potatoes).
- Avoid gas-producing, cruciferous vegetables: broccoli, cauliflower, Brussels sprouts, asparagus, onions, garlic, beans, and peas.
- Avoid carbonated beverages.
- Avoid excess sugar-free chewing gum or products containing sorbitol, mannitol, and xylitol.
- Avoid temperature extremes in foods.
- Avoid caffeine and alcohol.

Encourage the following foods:

- Pureed cooked fruit (applesauce), bananas, fruit canned in juice
- White rice
- Plain pasta
- Plain white toast
- Mashed or baked potatoes without skin
- Tapioca
- Oatmeal
- Cream of rice
- Saltines
- Baked chips
- Lean meats (beef, turkey, chicken, fish)
- Scrambled egg whites

- Boiled eggs
- Marshmallows
- Gingersnaps
- Pureed fruit pouches

Dysgeusia

Significant changes in taste can occur from oral mucosal cellular destruction and desensitization. Fortunately, changes in taste typically diminish over time once therapy has been completed. Olfactory changes may also occur, further exacerbating the displeasure associated with eating. Dysgeusia also contributes to nausea and food aversions. Helping patients cope with this side effect requires encouraging experimentation with new flavors and avoidance of unpleasant tastes and odors. The basic 5 tastes of sweetness, sourness, saltiness, bitterness, and umami (pleasant savory taste) are negatively affected and may become difficult to detect. Strategies to encourage and implement include[21]

- Encourage a trial of zinc supplementation. (Chronic losses from diarrhea may alter taste.)
- Encourage a trial of new flavors and spices, such as fresh or dried herbs. Crush mint leaves and add to water or tea.
- Encourage adding salt, soy sauce, and balsamic vinegar to foods.
- Encourage adding sauces to help moisten foods and add flavor.
- Encourage adding tart jams or jellies to fruit.
- Dilute juice and add lemon and lime slices to water.
- Encourage additional seasoning of meats with fruit or salty marinades or replace meats with eggs, yogurt, cheese sticks, smoothies, or flavored milk.
- Encourage eating foods cold or at room temperature.
- Encourage eating hard candy to offset having a bad taste in the mouth.
- Discourage drinking coffee and unflavored tea.

Xerostomia

Chemotherapy, medications, and radiation therapy to the head and neck may cause xerostomia making eating, swallowing, and even speaking unpleasant. Strategies to help your patients combat this symptom include[21]

- Encourage the use of sauces and gravies to soften and moisten foods.
- Discourage eating dry foods that may also be difficult to chew, such as bread, crackers, or unseasoned meats.
- Encourage eating soups and stews.
- Encourage eating pureed fruits, smoothies, and desserts between meals to increase calorie intake.
- Encourage eating sour hard candy or foods to help stimulate saliva production.

Mucositis and Pharyngitis

The oral mucosa is particularly susceptible to destruction during cancer therapy. Oral and throat inflammatory changes, lesions and ulcerations can make eating and swallowing painful and difficult for patients. The following strategies will help reduce oral pain and discomfort[21]:

- Encourage eating bland, soft, and moist foods.
- Encourage eating fluids, bland smoothies, soups and stews.
- Encourage the use of a straw if lip sores are present.

- Discourage eating dry, difficult-to-chew foods, such as bread, crackers, and nuts.
- Discourage eating acidic foods, such as citrus fruit, tomatoes, and pickled foods.
- Discourage eating spicy and salty foods.
- Encourage the addition of milk and condensed milk to foods.
- Encourage mashing or pureeing fruits and vegetable, such as potatoes, sweet potatoes, and carrots.
- Encourage adding canola, coconut, or olive oil to foods to help soften texture and increase calories.
- Encourage eating cooked cereal moistened with milk or condensed milk, such as oatmeal and cream of rice.
- Encourage eating protein-boosted puddings with added nonfat milk powder.
- Discourage the consumption of alcohol, carbonated beverages, or rough-textured foods.

MAINTENANCE AND PREVENTION

The completion of cancer treatment is a perfect time to continue educating your patients about the importance of nutrition. At this point, if oral intake and weight loss continue to be a challenge, many of the specialized nutrition support techniques described earlier should still be encouraged and used. However, if these issues no longer exist, then this is the perfect opportunity to begin the discussion of maintaining a healthy diet and healthy weight. It is important to remember that patients with cancer are particularly vulnerable to misinformation provided by well-intentioned caretakers and the multitude of online resources. Fad diets and unnecessary restrictions are not appropriate and can potentially cause harm. The discussions should focus on maintaining a healthy lifestyle. A registered dietitian and experienced strength and conditioning coach can assist with maintenance of a healthy lifestyle within safe medical parameters and guidelines set by the medical team. Some general guidelines include

- Eat a variety of healthy foods daily.
- Limit processed, fried, and fatty foods.
- Consume 2 to 3 cups of fruits and vegetables daily.
- Encourage eating whole grains, barley, oats, and quinoa.
- Increase the intake of fish and poultry and reduce red meats.
- Cook with olive oil.
- Encourage healthy cooking habits, such as baking, broiling, poaching, and grilling.
- Increase the intake of foods high in antioxidants and phytochemicals.
- Consume foods high in dietary fiber.
- Stay active.
- Encourage stretching and flexibility.
- Stay hydrated with healthy beverages, such as water, sports drinks, and coconut water.
- Limit alcohol intake.

SUMMARY/DISCUSSION

Cancer treatment results in various medical and social challenges, particularly in the area of nutrition. Individualizing patients' nutritional plan requires diligent daily monitoring and evaluation of clinical status, gastrointestinal function, laboratory values, intake and output, body weight, history and physical examination, therapies and medications, patient preferences, and prognosis. First-line medical providers can significantly improve the quality of life for patients with cancer by intervening early and often, building rapport, and implementing a daily process for individualizing nutrition support. Simply put, we must have nutrition to heal. Without adequate and appropriate nutrition, a positive outcome is just not possible.

REFERENCES

1. Ramos EJ, Suzuki S, Marks D, et al. Cancer anorexia-cachexia syndrome: cytokines and neuropeptides. Curr Opin Clin Nutr Metab Care 2004;7:427–34.
2. Davis MP, Dreicer R, Walsh D, et al. Appetite and cancer-associated anorexia: a review. J Clin Oncol 2004;22:1510–7.
3. Dahele M, Fearon KCH. Research methodology: cancer cachexia syndrome. Palliat Med 2004;18:409–17.
4. Tisdale MJ. Patogenesis of cancer cachexia. J Support Oncol 2003;1:159–68.
5. Shils ME, Shike M. Nutritional support of the cancer patient. In: Shils ME, Olson J, Shike M, et al, editors. Modern nutrition in health and disease. Baltimore (MD): Williams & Wilkins; 1999. p. 1297–325.
6. Gilbreath J, Inman-Felton A, Johnson EQ, et al. Medical nutrition therapy across the continuum of care-client protocols. 2nd edition. Chicago: The American Dietetic Association; 1998.
7. Hurst JD, Gallagher AL. Energy, macronutrient, micronutrient, and fluid requirements. In: Elliot L, Molseed LL, McCallum PD, editors. The clinical guide to oncology nutrition. 2nd edition. Chicago: The American Dietetic Association; 2006. p. 54–71.
8. Knox LS, Crosby LO, Feurer ID, et al. Energy expenditure in malnourished cancer patients. Ann Surg 1983;197:152–62.
9. Brown J, Byers T, Thompson K, et al, American Cancer Society Work group on Nutrition and Physical Activity for Cancer Survivors. Nutrition during and after cancer treatment: a guide for informed choices by cancer survivors. CA Cancer J Clin 2001;51:153–87.
10. Le RD, Nieman DC. Meauring diet. In: Lee RD, Nieman DC, editors. Nutritional assessment. 3rd edition. New York: McGraw-Hill; 2003. p. 73–110.
11. Russell MK. Nutrition screening and assessment. In: Gottschlich MM, editor. The A.S.P.E.N. Nutrition support core curriculum: a case-based approach – the adult patient. 2nd edition. ASPEN; 2007. p. 167–8, 170–1.
12. Wooley JA. Energy. In: Gottschlich MM, editor. The A.S.P.E.N. Nutrition support core curriculum: a case-based approach – the adult patient. 2nd edition. ASPEN; 2007. p. 20–7.
13. Hise ME. Lipids. In: Gottschlich MM, editor. The A.S.P.E.N. Nutrition support core curriculum: a case-based approach – the adult patient. 2nd edition. Patent; 2007. p. 56–8.
14. ASPEN Board of Directors and the Clinical Guidelines Task Force. Guidelines for the use of parenteral and enteral nutrition in adult and pediatric patients. JPEN J Parenter Enteral Nutr 2002;26(Suppl):1SA–137SA.
15. Jatoi A, Windschitl HE, Loprinzi CL, et al. Dronabinol versus megestrol acetate versus combination therapy for cancer-associated anorexia: a north centeral cancer treatment group study. J Clin Oncol 2002;20:567–73.
16. Woolridge JE, Anderson CM, Perry MC. Corticosteroids in advanced cancer. Oncology 2001;15:225–36.

17. Muscaritoli M, Bossola M, Bellantone R, et al. Therapy of muscle wasting in cancer: what is the future? Curr Opin Clin Nutr Metab Care 2004;7:459–66.

18. Eder U, Mangweth B, Ebenbichler C, et al. Association of olanzapine-induced weight gain with an increase in body fat. Am J Psychiatry 2001; 158:1719–22.

19. Dewys WD, Begg C, Lavin PT, et al. Prognostic effect of weight loss prior to chemotherapy in cancer patients. Am J Med 1989;68:491–7.

20. Bosaeus I, Daneryd P, Lundholm K. Dietary intake, resting energy expenditure, weight loss and survival in cancer patients. J Nutr 2002;132(Suppl 11): 3465S–6S.

21. Robert S, Thompson J. Graft-vs-host disease: nutrition therapy in a challenging condition. Nutr Clin Pract 2005;20:440–50.

Oncology: Symptom Management

Ian Nagus, PA-C, MS[a],*, Courtney Moller, PA-C, MS[b]

KEYWORDS

- Symptom • Palliative care • Assessment • Pain • Side effects

KEY POINTS

- Developing an understanding of typical symptoms, and an approach to treating them, is of paramount importance to oncology providers.
- Palliative or supportive care specialists have been proved to improve patient outcomes when mobilized for the care of oncology patients.
- In order to best alleviate a particular symptom, clinicians must first understand its cause, and then mobilize both pharmacologic and nonpharmacologic treatments specific to that individual.

INTRODUCTION

Over the next 15 years, the percentage of the US population more than 65 years of age will continue to grow. Roughly 1 out of every 5 Americans will fit into this aging demographic. Although this time of life can be associated with increased independence, financial security, and good health, it is also a time associated with possible functional decline and physical/psychosocial distress related to chronic and advanced illness.[1]

The awareness and continued growth of palliative medicine as a specialty has better prepared clinicians to deal with the unique medical challenges anticipated to affect the aging population. As the age of the population increases, so will the incidence and prevalence of cancer. More than 1.5 million new cancer diagnoses were made in the United States in 2015. The US medical system must improve past the current limitations of medical care. One of the most common challenges to date has been the undertreatment of symptoms.[2] By using routine assessments, clinicians can make progress to identify overlooked and unreported symptoms, facilitate treatment, and enhance patient and family satisfaction.[3]

This article presents the concept of palliative care, describes the principles of symptom management, and provides examples of potential treatment options for these common complaints specific to patients living with a cancer diagnosis.

Disclosures: None.
[a] Mass General/North Shore Cancer Center, 102 Endicott Street, Danvers, MA 01923, USA;
[b] Dana Farber Cancer Institute, 450 Brookline Avenue, Boston, MA 02115, USA
* Corresponding author.
E-mail address: inagus@partners.org

Physician Assist Clin 1 (2016) 375–395
http://dx.doi.org/10.1016/j.cpha.2016.03.011
2405-7991/16/$ – see front matter © 2016 Elsevier Inc. All rights reserved.

PALLIATIVE CARE

Palliative care is a practice both old and new to medicine. It is old in terms of its concept and ideals, but fairly new in its recognition as a formal specialty. The term was initially coined in the 1970s by Balfour Mount to describe a Canadian medical program that was based on the hospice model. A strategy of treatment focusing on symptom management (not curing a disease) was popular long before the first official hospice facility opened in London in 1967, and in the United States in 1975.[4] In some centers across the country, it is also referred to as supportive care.

In recent years, several organizations have attempted to define palliative care. These simple definitions have often been limited and have failed to describe the totality of the specialty.[5,6] As the field has emerged, more suitable definitions have been offered:

Palliative care is specialized medical care for people with serious illnesses. This type of care is focused on providing patients with relief from the symptoms, pain, and stress of serious illness. The goal is to improve quality of life for both the patient and the family. Palliative care is provided by a team of doctors, nurses and other specialists who work with a patient's other doctors to provide an extra layer of support. Palliative care is appropriate at any age and at any stage in a serious illness, and can be provided together with curative treatment.[6]

Frequently and incorrectly, palliative care is thought to be equivalent to end of life or hospice care. The main difference between these two types of care is that palliative care can be offered to a much wider population of patients. It can be used at any time, for any patient. In contrast, in order to qualify for hospice care, the patient must be living with a life-limiting illness, and have a prognosis limited to 6 months or less. Many patients, even early in disease states (whether curable or not), have physical, psychosocial, and spiritual symptoms and distress that can be addressed and improved through palliative-care support.

Interdisciplinary Approach

Although most specialties in medicine focus on a specific organ system or problem, palliative-care teams are able to provide comprehensive care if there are complex and serious medical issues. They are able to provide this global care because palliative medicine is practiced as an interdisciplinary team. Teams are often inclusive of clinicians (physicians, physician assistants, nurse practitioners), palliative care–trained nurses, social workers, chaplains, and pharmacists. Reviews of many studies suggest that this approach results in benefits to patients and their families, as well as to the health care system. Some data include, but are but not limited to, improved patient/family satisfaction, reduced hospital costs, improved symptom management, and increased likelihood that patient die in their own homes.[7]

Palliative Care in Oncology

Many symptoms experienced by oncology patients are related to the effect of the disease burden, or immediate reactions to treatments (surgery, chemotherapy, hormonal therapy, immunotherapy, radiation). Common symptoms that are experienced include pain, dyspnea, nausea and vomiting, constipation, diarrhea, fatigue, mood changes, delirium, and skin changes. When palliative care is initiated early, patients and families can be supported throughout the course of illness. The palliative-care team also can support oncologists in the mutual care of patients.

Because many patients achieve a period of remission or cure, they can experience long-lasting permanent symptoms related to the initial disease. Their symptoms need to continue to be addressed through palliative care or in survivorship clinics. Examples of these types of symptoms include chronic pain, neuropathy, dysphagia, and psychosocial distress (anxiety, depression).

Benefits of Early Palliative Care

Recent research has highlighted what palliative-care practitioners have known for years; that palliative care not only improves quality of life but can help people live longer. A 2010 Massachusetts General Hospital study reported on a group of patients with stage IV non–small cell lung cancer. These patients were randomized to receive standard oncologic care or standard oncologic care plus early palliative care. The outcomes revealed that early palliative care helped improve both the quality of life and the mood of patients, in addition to preventing less aggressive care at end of life, and prolonged survival rate by about 2 months.[5] This study and others have led organizations like the American Organization of Clinical Oncology and the American Society of Medical Oncology to suggest that early palliative care should now be the gold standard in patients with advanced disease.[8]

When a Palliative-Care Team Is Not Available

Significant increases have been made in the availability of palliative-care programs across the United States. In 2015, there are palliative-care experts available in 67% of US hospitals.[9] That leaves a gap of one-third of hospitals that do not have this support available to their patients or staff. Through formal training programs and online resources, it is now possible for all medical providers to complement their skill sets and improve the experience of their patients. The Center to Advance Palliative Care is one of several national organizations dedicated to increasing the availability of quality palliative-care services for people facing serious illness. This organization has led the cultural transformation of this medical subspecialty across the globe, and has consistently been a leader in providing both provider and patient resources for support. Through the use of their articles, videos, podcasts, training programs, and fast facts, any clinician can be empowered to provide expert symptom management.[10]

The effects of living with a cancer diagnosis are multidimensional. Sequelae of the disease and its treatment can vary, even among patients with common cancer types and receiving similar treatments. These effects can fundamentally influence the body, mind, and spirit. With or without access to expert palliative care, the responsibility of providers is to anticipate effects, guide their patients, and mobilize strategies to best support patients as they live with a cancer diagnosis. The most important tool any clinician can have is the awareness to routinely ask patients about their side effects and listen to their concerns, even if they are not apparent, when they walk into the examination room.

SYMPTOM MANAGEMENT: COMMON APPROACH

In an effort to provide consistent and thorough care of patients, many clinicians use a simple framework to organize the process of assessment and treatment. Several common tools include the use of mnemonic devices, surveys, and checklists. The information gleaned from these tools, coupled with thorough physical examination and appropriate diagnostic testing, leads to a presumed diagnosis and a thoughtful assessment and plan.

Interview

Two mnemonic devices and several assessment tools are offered later as a basic framework to support practices when interviewing patients about their symptoms.

One of the most well-known mnemonic devices used by medical professionals to accurately discern history in the event of acute illness or understanding of symptoms has been the alphabetical run of MOPQRST. Many clinicians were provided this clinical pearl in their training, and use this tool frequently. This mnemonic has been further adapted in emergency situations to elicit symptoms of a possible heart attack[11] and in palliative medicine to ascribe meaning and definition to symptoms.[12]

Each consecutive letter represents a line of specific questioning designed to provide the most accurate and appropriate assessment of the situation or symptom experienced:

M: meaning of a symptom to the patient (psychosocial connection)
O: onset (acute vs chronic)
P: provoking factors and palliating factors
Q: quality of symptom (description of what it feels like)
R: related; factors/symptoms (associated symptoms; physical/psychological)
S: severity (rating)
T: temporality/timing (when did it start/how long does it last)

Symptom-Rating Instruments

Although it is time consuming, it is critically important to obtain the severity rating of a patient's symptoms frequently. This practice establishes a baseline understanding of distress and acts as a guide to adjust the therapeutic plan. Most clinicians are familiar with using a symptom-rating scale when evaluating pain. These scales most often use a verbal, numerical, or visual analog scale and many can be used in both the adult and pediatric populations. These approaches are based on studies in subjective sensory physiology, in which it has been shown that perception of a stimulus is closely related to the strength of the stimulus.[13]

An alternative approach to the use of standard analog scales is to use descriptive responses. Such responses might be: not effected, bothers me a little bit, somewhat, quite a bit, very much, and so forth. These defined responses may be more helpful with specific symptoms that are harder to quantify, such as fatigue. Examples of these types of scales are Eastern Cooperative Oncology Group Performance Status, Karnofsky Performance Scale, and the Palliative Performance Scale. Another way to show symptom severity and provide another means of monitoring therapeutic outcomes is to ask patients to quantify and describe how symptoms affect their daily activities.[14]

Several validated multiple symptom assessment tools are in wide usage and may prove useful to supporting practices. A list of several of the most commonly used is given here.

- The Edmonton Symptom Assessment Scale[15]
- Memorial Symptom Assessment Scale–Short[16]
- MD Anderson Brief Symptom Inventory[17]
- Rotterdam Symptom Checklist[18]
- Symptom Distress Scale[19]
- The National Comprehensive Cancer Network Distress Thermometer[20]

Assessment

It is in understanding the dimensions of a symptom, and matching them with objective measures of history, vital signs, medication administration, and diagnostic testing, that clinicians can begin to formulate a likely diagnosis. Once a diagnosis has been made for any particular malady or symptom, then comes the hard part: improving it.

Treatment

A common and simple strategy often used for the treatment of symptoms can be thought of in 4 parts and can be remembered with another mnemonic device. Common symptoms and treatment pearls for each are highlighted later.

  T: treat reversible causes
  O: optimize pharmaceutical treatment
  N: nonpharmacologic support of symptoms
  I: invasive procedures

PHYSICAL SYMPTOMS
Pain

Control of cancer-related pain is achievable by simple means in 75% to 90% of patients.[21] In order to relieve suffering in this percentage of patients, it is imperative that clinicians understand their pain. Pain should not be solely appreciated by a relative rating score of 0 to 10, and it should not be treated uniformly with a narcotic.

When treating pharmacologically, it is particularly important to remember that analgesic side effects require prophylaxis, early recognition, and aggressive intervention. If systemic analgesics and nonpharmacologic interventions are ineffective, or produce intolerable side effects, then clinicians should also consider interventional analgesic options.

Understand and treat the specific cause:

The most effective way to manage pain is to remove the cause. To understand the process driving the symptom, clinicians must be diligent in their interview technique and diagnostic approach. Taking a thorough medical history and eliciting an adequate pain assessment are the keys to determining the source of pain, and its most effective treatment options. Once the components of a pain history, medical history, and diagnostic testing are all integrated, then it is hoped that the outcome will lead to a specific pain diagnosis.

An example of mnemonic device (PAINED) used to help guide clinicians in performing a pain history.

Place: where is the pain? Can it be pointed to or is it in a general area?
Amount: rate it on scale, and how long has it been present?
Intensifiers: what makes it worse?
Nullifiers: what makes it better?
Effects: what is the effect of analgesics/what is the effect on quality of life?
Description: describe how it feels (stabbing, aching, burning, and so forth)?

Once the cause of the pain is understood in the context of the symptoms, then occasionally simple solutions can be used. Quick solutions could be antibiotics prescribed for a superficial infections, or removal of fluids for ascites or effusions.

Common causes of cancer-related pain include but are not limited to:

- Metastatic disease in organs, soft tissues, bone, muscle, central nervous system
- Infection

- Mucositis
- Pathologic fracture
- Treatment-associated neuropathy
- Psychosomatic manifestation of pain

Fig. 1 shows an example of a single presenting complaint related to metastatic disease and how different pain syndromes can be described from a common finding of vertebral metastases. Each pain syndrome is different, and thus is treated uniquely.

Optimize analgesics and adjuvant medications

Because the mainstay of treating pain is with pharmacotherapy it is important to become familiar with the available medication options. Clinicians must become aware of the relative benefits and burdens of each analgesic. Opioids, antiinflammatories, anticonvulsants, selective serotonin reuptake inhibitors (SSRI)/serotonin norepinephrine reuptake inhibitors (SNRIs), and bisphosphonates are the most common medications typically considered. Once clinicians understand the potential side effect profiles of these drug classes, then they can think proactively and act aggressively in limiting the negative effect. The most common example of this is initiating laxatives for an individual requiring opioid therapy. It is understood that the most common side effect of using narcotic pain medicine is slow-transit constipation.

Table 1 lists common pain syndromes and therapeutic options for these.

The World Health Organization (WHO) has developed a 3-step ladder for pharmacologic management of cancer pain.[22] Every clinician should be aware of this strategic recommendation and its rationale (**Fig. 2**).

The concept of this ladder is to encourage clinicians to administer analgesics for cancer-related pain in the following order: nonopioids (aspirin and paracetamol); then, as necessary, mild opioids (codeine); then strong opioids such as morphine, until the patient is free of pain. The secondary suggestion is to be mindful of and treat fears and anxiety, with additional drugs (adjuvants) as needed. Use of the different medication options provides better analgesia than any single class of medication alone.[21] In the case of cancer pain in children, WHO recommends a 2-step ladder.[22]

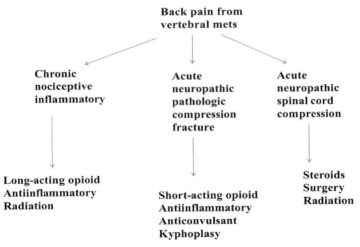

Fig. 1. A single presenting complaint related to metastatic disease (mets).

Table 1
Common pain syndromes and therapeutic options

Type of Pain	Adjuvant Type	Analgesic
Bone pain	Bisphosphonates	Pamidronate/zoledronic acid
	Radiation	Targeted therapy/injected radiopharmaceutical
	NSAIDs	Naproxen/acetaminophen/ketorolac
	Steroids	Systemic/local: injected
Neuropathic pain	Anticonvulsants	Gabapentin/pregabalin
	Tricyclic antidepressants	Nortryptyline/amytriptyline
	SNRI/SSRI	Duloxetine/venlafaxine
	Local anesthetic	Lidocaine patch/capsacin
Inflammatory pain	NSAIDs	Naproxen/acetaminophen/ketorolac
	Steroids	Systemic/local: injected
Mucositis	Mouthwash (nonalcohol)	Biotene
	Local anesthetics	Magic mouthwash: viscous lidocaine
	NSAIDs	Ketorolac
	Steroids	Systemic
	PPI/H2 antagonist	Omeprazole/famotidine
Malignant wounds	Antibiotics	Specific to cultured bacteria
	Topical opioid	Morphine: intrasite gel
	NSAID	Naproxen/acetaminophen/ketorolac

Abbreviations: NSAIDs, nonsteroidal antiinflammatory drugs; PPI, proton pump inhibitor.

Nonpharmacologic interventions

When considering a treatment of cancer-related pain, it is important to consider that patients' functional goals are best achieved by combining adequate analgesia with rehabilitative therapies (physical therapy, occupational therapy).[23] Reaching out to colleagues in these disciplines for support is of great benefit to patients.

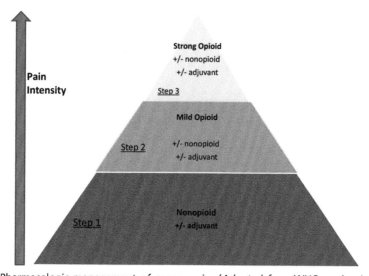

Fig. 2. Pharmacologic management of cancer pain. (*Adapted from* WHO analgesic ladder. Available at: http://www.who.int/cancer/palliative/painladder/en/. Accessed December 9, 2015.)

The addition of psychosocial and spiritual support coupled with integrative therapies can also aid in alleviating pain and suffering. As clinicians try to identify all possible allies in helping to treat the pain and limit narcotics, it is important to ask each patient about any past beneficial experiences.

A list of common nonpharmacologic options that have been reported to help relieve suffering associated with unrelenting pain is presented later (**Table 2**). When used as preventive strategies, or during a pain crisis, these simple strategies can make a significant difference[23]:

Psychological counseling
Stretching/positioning

Table 2
Dyspnea: pharmacologic and nonpharmacologic interventions

Cause	Pharmacologic Treatment	Nonpharmacologic Treatment
Pleural effusion[24,25]	Opioids: PO, IV, or SQ dose determined when symptoms relieved	• Thoracentesis • Pleura drain placement • Pleurodesis • Thoracoscopy
Reactive airway/ bronchospasm[24,26]	• Steroids • Albuterol • Ipratropium • Opioids: PO, IV, SQ, or nebulized[24]	• Bedside fan • Supplemental O_2
Primary or metastatic disease in lung[24]	• Chemotherapy • Opioids: PO, IV, or SQ • Benzodiazepine: PO or IV	• Radiation therapy • Surgical resection • Bedside fan • Supplemental O_2
Pulmonary emboli	• Anticoagulation • Discontinuing any medication that may increase risk of emboli	• Bedside fan • Supplemental O_2
Airway obstruction[24,26]	• Steroids • Opioids: PO, IV, or SQ	• Radiation therapy • Bronchial stenting • Supplemental O_2 • Supplemental O_2 with helium
Ischemic heart disease	• Opioids: IV, SQ • Nitroglycerin • Aspirin • β-Blockers	• Supplemental O_2 • Cardiac catheterization
Pericardial disease/effusion	• Opioids: PO, IV, or SQ • Corticosteroids: for pericarditis	• Pericardiocentesis • Pericardial window • Supplemental O_2
Heart failure	• ACE-I/ARB • β-Blockers • Diuresis • Opioids: PO, IV, SQ	Supplemental O_2
Anemia[24,26]	• Erythropoietin • Darbepoietin	• Blood transfusion • Supplemental O_2
Anxiety	Benzodiazepines: PO, IV	• Breathing exercises • Meditation • Supplemental O_2

Abbreviations: ACE-I, angiotensin-converting enzyme inhibitors; ARB, angiotensin receptor blockers; IV, intravenous; PO, by mouth; SQ, subcutaneous.

Ice/heat
Splinting
Meditation/yoga/deep breathing
Acupuncture
Guided imagery
Reiki
Massage

Invasive interventions
Some form of invasive intervention is needed by 10% of patients with cancer-related pain.[21] Often these interventions are used when systemic pharmacotherapy has failed or the side effects of the analgesics are self-limiting. Nerve blocks, ablations, and intraspinal analgesics may enhance pain control with fewer systemic side effects. With these interventions the problem is being treated locally and the medications can be delivered at a smaller dose than is required with systemic therapy.[27]

A list of common types interventional analgesic strategies used for specific types of cancer pain is presented here:

Celiac plexus block: pancreatic or gastric cancer pain
Kyphoplasty: pathologic compression fractures compressing nerves
Epidural steroid injection: neuropathic cancer pain from tumor
Epidural/intrathecal pump placement: refractory pain with high incidence of side effects from systemic analgesics

Dyspnea

Dyspnea is a common symptom among patients with cancer. Estimates of those affected range from 20% to 90%. Those typically affected tend to have either primary or metastatic disease involving their lungs; however, those without disease in their lungs can also experience dyspnea.[26]

Dyspnea is mediated by 4 possible different pathophysiologic pathways[24]:

1. Receptors at alveoli and capillaries that respond to fluid and microemboli
2. Mechanoreceptors that react based on stretch in lungs, airways, or chest
3. Chemoreceptors that respond to hypoxia in aorta and carotid bodies
4. Chemoreceptors that respond to CO_2

Common causes
Pulmonary:
- Pleural effusion
- Reactive airway/bronchospasm
- Primary or metastatic disease to lung
- Pulmonary emboli
- Airway obstruction

Cardiac:
- Ischemic heart disease
- Pericardial disease or effusion
- Heart failure
- Superior vena cava syndrome
- Anemia

Psychosocial:
- Anxiety

Opioid dosing

- Opioid-naive patient: start low dose and titrate up for effect (ie, 7.5–15 mg morphine by mouth, or 2–5 mg intravenously)[25]
- If the patient is already on opioids, increase dose by 25% and titrate for effect
- All opioids can be used effectively for dyspnea

Benzodiazepine dosing

- Lorazepam 0.5 mg every 4 hours as needed, by mouth, subcutaneously, or intravenously[25]

Nausea and Vomiting

Nausea and vomiting remain among the most common side effects of cancer and its treatments, and are the side effects that many patients associate with the word cancer. Nausea is the sensation that normally precedes the act of vomiting. Nausea and vomiting occur after stimulation of one of the following sites: gastrointestinal tract, the chemoreceptor trigger zone, the central nervous system, or the vestibular system.[28] As noted with other symptoms, getting an accurate and detailed history of the symptom helps in determining the most appropriate and effective treatment (**Table 3**).

Common causes

Gastrointestinal tract:
- Gastroesophageal reflux disease
- Constipation/gastroparesis
- Obstruction
- Infection

Chemoreceptor zone (chemical/metabolic):
- Toxins (metabolic)
- Medications: chemotherapies and opioids

Central nervous system:
- Increased intracranial pressure
- New or worsening brain metastasis
- Psychoemotional: anxiety

Vestibular:
- Motion sickness
- Movement-related vomiting or nausea

Nonpharmacologic interventions

- Suggest patients eat smaller more frequent meals[29]
- Have patients and caregivers avoid food that smells unpleasant to the patient
- Suggest that patients practice relaxation techniques around mealtime
- Consider alternative therapies, such as hypnosis, acupuncture, reiki
- Consider surgical evaluation for management of obstruction, and consideration of nasogastric tube decompression, resection, stenting, or venting gastric tube

Constipation

Constipation is described as limited amount or frequency of stool that causes discomfort. A normal bowel pattern is considered to be at least 3 bowel movements per week, but fewer than 3 a day[30] (**Table 4**).

Table 3
Nausea and vomiting pharmacologic interventions

Cause	Type of Nausea/ Vomiting	Pharmacologic Treatment Options
Increased gastric acidity or GERD	Gastrointestinal	• PPI (like omeprazole) BID and/or • H2 blocker (like famotidine) BID
Constipation	Gastrointestinal	(See text) • Bowel softeners, laxatives, enemas, suppositories
Gastroparesis	Gastrointestinal	Reglan 5–10 mg TID–QID
Obstruction (SBO, colonic obstruction, peritoneal carcinomatosis, mass effect)	Gastrointestinal	• Octreotide 100—200 µg SQ/IV BID–TID • Dexamethasone 4–10 mg IV or PO BID (can also be given PRN) • Maximize constipation regimen
Infection	Gastrointestinal	Treat underlying infection with appropriate antibiotic course
Medication: chemotherapy	Chemoreceptor zone	• Zofran 4–8 mg IV/PO BID–TID • Compazine 5–10 mg IV/PP TID–QID (can also be given PRN) • Emend 125 mg PO before chemotherapy, then 80 mg PO QAM × 2 d
Medication: opioids	Chemoreceptor zone	• Zofran 4–8 mg IV/PO BID–TID • Compazine 5–10 mg IV/PO TID–QID • Haldol 0.5-1 mg IV/PO BID–TID • Zyprexa/Zydis 2.5–5 mg PO/SL QD–BID
Electrolyte abnormalities (ie, uremia, hypercalcemia)	Chemoreceptor zone	• Treat the underlying abnormality if possible • Zofran 4–8 mg IV/PO BID–TID • Compazine 5–10 mg IV/PO TID–QID • Haldol 0.5–1 mg IV/PO BID–TID • Zyprexa/Zydis 2.5–5 mg PO/SL QD–BID • Marinol 2.5–10 mg PO QD
Brain metastasis or primary tumor	Central nervous system	Dexamethasone 4–10 mg IV or PO BID
Anxiety or psychoemotional	Central nervous system	Lorazepam 0.5–2 mg IV/PO/SL q 4–6 h PRN
Motion sickness (positional nausea/ vomiting)	Vestibular	• Scopolamine 1.5 mg patch TD q 72 h • Meclizine 25–50 mg PO BID • Levsin 1–2 tsp (solution) or 1–2 tab q 4 h PRN

Abbreviations: BID, twice a day; GERD, gastroesophageal reflux disease; PRN, as needed; QAM, every morning; QD, every day; q, every; QID, 4 times a day; SBO, small bowel obstruction; SL, sublingual; tab, tablets; TD, total dose; TID, 3 times a day; tsp, teaspoons.

From Abrahm J. Physician's guide to pain and symptom management in cancer patients. Baltimore (MD): The Johns Hopkins University Press; 2014. p. 450–60; with permission.

Common causes

- Medications: opioids, chemotherapy (vinca alkaloids, oxaliplatins, taxanes, and thalidomide), calcium-based and aluminum-based antacids, diuretics, vitamins, and anticholinergics[30]
- Change in motility: prolonged immobilization
- Neuromuscular disorders: spinal cord injury and paraplegia
- Environmental factors: change in bathroom habits, inability to get to bathroom
- Narrowing of the colon lumen related to tumor, effects of radiation treatment

Table 4
Constipation-pharmacologic interventions

Laxatives	
Stimulants: work by increasing enteric muscle contraction and GI motility.[31] Onset is 6–12 h	• Senna 2 tab QHS–BID • Bisacodyl 10 mg PO or 10 mg PRN QD–BID
Osmotic: work by increasing colonic intraluminal water through oncotic pressure.[31] Onset is 12–48 h	• MiraLax 17 g PO QD–BID • Lactulose 15–30 g QD
Saline: high osmolarity draws water into lumen of intestine.[30] Onset 0.5–3 h	• Magnesium sulfate 15 g QD • Milk of magnesia 15–30 mL QD PRN • Magnesium citrate 240 mL QD PRN
Lubricant: lubricate intestinal mucosa and soften stool[30]	Mineral oil PO 5–30 mL QHS
Stool Softeners	
Encourage water retention in fecal mass. It can take several days before effect is seen. In general, used in combination with 1 or more of the above laxatives[30]	Docusate 100–300 mg PO QD until BM is normal

Abbreviations: BM, bowel movement; GI, gastrointestinal; QHS, at bedtime.

Enemas:
- Mineral oil print rectum, followed by soap suds: mineral oil is given first to soften the stool, followed by soap suds to induce peristalsis.
- Tap water enema.
- Milk and molasses: combine equal parts molasses (235 mL [8 oz]) and milk (235 mL), warmed together and then hung in an enema bag. This mixture is thought to increase peristalsis and be gentle on the lining of the colon.

Opioid antagonists:
- Methylnaltrexone 0.15 mg/kg daily or every other day for opioid-induced constipation[30]
  - Cannot be given safely in patients with bowel obstructions
  - Should only be given once other modalities have failed

Nonpharmacologic interventions

- Encourage physical activity[32]
- Obtain private setting for toileting[32]
- Encourage increased fluid intake
- Encourage fiber intake
- Provide warm drink about 30 minutes before usual toileting time[30]

Diarrhea

Diarrhea is another common gastrointestinal symptom for many patients with cancer. Diarrhea is described as abnormal looseness of stools with increased liquidity or decreased consistency.[33] It can be graded on a scale of 1 to 4 in severity based on the number of increased stools per day, and how it affects the patient's functioning (**Tables 5** and **6**).[35]

Table 5
National Cancer Institute's common terminology criteria for adverse events: diarrhea

Grade	Description
1	Mild increase in output compared with baseline. Increase of <4 stools day
2	Increase of 4–6 stools over baseline; moderate increase in output compared with baseline
3	Increase >7 stools/d over baseline, ± incontinence. Hospitalization indicated. Severe increase in ostomy output compared with baseline, limiting self-care/ADLs
4	Life-threatening consequences. Urgent intervention indicated
5	Death

Abbreviation: ADLs, activities of daily living.

Common causes

Cancer-related treatment[35]

- Chemotherapy: most commonly therapies containing irinotecan or fluoropyrimidines
- Radiation: causing radiation enteritis
- Surgery: changing structure of gastrointestinal tract (or surrounding structures)
- Bone marrow transplant: commonly related to graft-versus-host disease (GVHD)
- Infectious: common infections for patients with cancer include *Clostridium difficile*

Medications[35]

- Antibiotics
- Overly aggressive bowel regimen
- Promotility agents (eg, Reglan, erythromycin)
- Cancer related: common symptom of colon cancer, lymphoma, or neuroendocrine tumors
- Fecal impaction: diarrhea can pass around impaction, and it may be the only stool that can pass through

Table 6
Diarrhea pharmacologic interventions

Type of Medication	Example
Opioid: reduces movement of gut, thereby reducing transit time[33]	Loperamide 4 mg, followed by 2 mg for each unformed stool thereafter. Maximum dose of 16 mg/d[34]
Antisecretory: inhibit mucosal prostaglandins[35]	• Octreotide 150–300 µg BID–TID or infused hourly over 24 h[34] (helpful in neuroendocrine tumors) • Aspirin: for radiation enteritis • Bismuth subsalicylate: can be added for increased symptoms related to *Escherichia coli* infection[33] • Corticosteroids: effective to reduce edema related to obstruction, and radiation effects
Antibiotics	As appropriate to treat the identified bacterial infection
Antiinflammatory	• Mesalamine: for inflammatory bowel disease[35] • Corticosteroids: effective to reduce edema related to obstruction, and radiation effects

Diet
- Products containing caffeine
- High-fiber diet
- Large amounts of lactose-containing foods, spicy foods, or gas-forming stools

Nonpharmacologic interventions

- Diet: recommended that patients eat a diet that is low in fiber, contains minerals, and is not irritating (ie, spicy foods, high-lactose foods, caffeine, alcohol, and fruit juices). Patients with mild diarrhea are recommended to follow the BRAT (bananas, rice, applesauce, toast) diet to reduce the number of stools.[35]
- Hydration: key to diarrhea treatment should be addressing the patient's fluid balance and extent of dehydration. The recommendation is that fluid intake be increased to 3 L/d during periods of diarrhea.
- Bowel rest: in patients in whom GVHD is suspected or obstruction, it is often recommended that the person has complete bowel rest for a period of time.[34]

Cancer-Related Fatigue

Fatigue is a prevalent symptom in patients with cancer, and it is exacerbated by often being under-recognized or its effects minimized because of the need to care for more painful or debilitating symptoms. Cancer-related fatigue is defined as a feeling of tiredness, and a lack of energy that is related to cancer and/or its treatments. It generally causes a change in functional ability and quality of life and is not relieved by rest.[36] It may be a symptom that patients often do not bring up on their own; however, when asked by a clinician, patients may welcome any advice on how to lessen fatigue's impact on their quality of life.

Common causes

Physiologic:
- Anemia
- Hypoxemia
- Cachexia
- Tumor burden
- Uncontrolled symptoms
- Electrolyte abnormalities

Behavioral:
- Change in functional status

Biochemical:
- Increased cytokine release
- Direct effects from cancer/treatment
- Sedating medications

Psychological:
- Depression
- Anxiety
- Difficulty sleeping

Pharmacologic interventions

The mainstay of pharmacologic treatments for cancer-related fatigue is psychostimulants; these include methylphenidate and modafinil. Although there remains a lack of good controlled studies for these drugs, there are some small studies that have shown efficacy. One such study evaluated 11 patients with advanced cancer and reports of fatigue, and found that 9 had improvement in reported fatigue with methylphenidate.[37] Another review found that methylphenidate improved opioid-induced somnolence as well as cognitive function when used in a palliative setting for treatment of depression.[38]

Additional treatment options include corticosteroids and megestrol. The beneficial effect of steroids always needs to be weighed against the possible side effects or toxicity. Megestrol is indicated with cancer-related cachexia when the possible benefits outweigh the increased risk of thromboembolism.[39] Other pharmacologic treatments may be intended to reverse any reversible causes (eg, treatment of other cancer-related symptoms, elimination of sedating drugs, treatment of anemia or electrolyte imbalances, and treatment of possible infections).

Nonpharmacologic interventions

- Normalization/education for patients and caregivers about cancer-related fatigue and setting realistic expectations for improved adaptation and adjustment of this symptom.
- Education regarding energy conservation and assistance in prioritizing activities and using techniques that protect the patient from physical and cognitive strain.
- Aerobic exercise has also shown benefit in management of cancer-related fatigue.[40] Specifically, clinicians should recommend moderate-intensity exercise that is progressive over time.

Pruritus

Pruritus is a common symptom in cancer, and can be related to the cancer itself, its treatments, or it may be unrelated.

Common causes

- Skin infections[41]
- Allergic reactions (to drugs [eg, chemotherapy, opioids, steroids] or otherwise)
- Metabolic (renal failure or liver failure)
- Disturbance of skin (eczema, radiation changes, irritation, chronic skin conditions)
- Cancer-induced pruritus (lymphoma, leukemia, polycythemia, iron deficiency)

Pharmacologic interventions

The most common pharmacologic treatments for pruritus include antihistamines and topical steroid preparations. In cases that do not respond to antihistamines or topical steroids, often a short course of systemic steroids is helpful. Other pharmacologic interventions include SSRIs/SNRIs, removal of offending agent or drug (most commonly chemotherapy or opioids), treatment of skin infection, and treatment of cancer.[42]

Nonpharmacologic interventions

The mainstay and first step in treatment of pruritus should be nonpharmacologic interventions. They include[42]:

- Avoiding hot showers/baths
- Using moisturizing emollients
- Using mild soaps and detergents
- Keeping environment cool and humid
- Oatmeal bath
- Stress reduction

PSYCHOSOCIAL CONCERNS

Individuals who have been diagnosed with cancer are particularly susceptible to increased psychosocial and emotional stress throughout the course of their lives after diagnosis. Symptoms may appear years after the malignancy has been treated.[43] Individuals may experience new and unique thoughts and feelings that influence how they are able to function within their family, community, or vocation. People affected by cancer might feel a general loss of control, and have to manage changes in coping and self-image. They might experience grief when considering their own physical losses and potential losses ahead.

It is the job of clinicians to identify these concerns early, and help provide a framework for support. Asking simple screening questions can often suffice to become aware of mood disorders like depression or anxiety (eg, asking whether the patient feels depressed/anxious). There are many screening tools that are more formal that also can guide clinicians to refer patients to seek out the counsel of a psychosocial specialist.

The importance of increasing the collective awareness of nonphysical symptoms is has merit. Previous data have shown that a lower quality of life and depressed mood are associated with shorter survival among patients with metastatic non–small cell lung cancer.[43–45] Interview-defined mood disorders have been shown to occur in roughly 30% to 40% of patients in hospital settings without a significant difference between palliative-care and non–palliative-care settings.[46] In follow-up care it is important to screen patients for these disorders, provide supportive care, and empower patients with information and self-management strategies.[47]

Of these mood disturbances, a diagnosis of adjustment disorder is common. An adjustment disorder can be characterized by inability to adjust to or cope with a particular stress or a major life event. The symptoms occur within 3 months of a major stressor and mimic those of clinical depression, such as general loss of interest, feelings of hopelessness, and crying.[48] It is sometimes known as situational depression. Unlike major depression, the disorder is caused by an outside stressor, generally resolves once the individual is able to adapt to the situation, and does not last longer than 6 months.

Depression

In general populations, the initial treatment of unipolar major depression is some combination of pharmacotherapy plus psychotherapy. Several classes of antidepressants are available and show comparable efficacy across and within classes. Choosing a drug is thus based on other factors (eg, drug delivery, side effect profile, and potential drug-drug interactions). Commonly SSRIs are the drugs of choice in the oncology population.

When initiating pharmacotherapy with antidepressants, there are a few clinical pearls to recall:

- Start at low doses and gradually up titrate over time
- Improvement is rarely immediate; counsel patients that it may take up to 2 weeks to appreciate the benefit
- If swallowing difficulties are anticipated, then consider an antidepressant that is available in liquid form

In combination with pharmacotherapy, several psychotherapies are available to treat major depression:

- Cognitive behavior therapy (CBT)
- Interpersonal psychotherapy

- Behavioral activation
- Family and couples therapy
- Problem-solving therapy
- Psychodynamic psychotherapy
- Supportive psychotherapy

Anxiety

As with treatment of individuals living with generalized anxiety disorder, it is common to take a 2-tiered approach to dealing with symptoms. On the first level clinicians may suggest using SSRIs or SNRIs and/or CBT. These efforts are mobilized to stabilize the mood and limit panic attacks. The second level of treatment commonly used, when the first level is ineffective, include SSRIs/SNRIs/tricyclic antidepressants/benzodiazepines, and anticonvulsants.[49]

Benzodiazepines are effective for acute and long-term treatment of anxiety, but clinicians should be wary of prescribing them to patients with a history of substance abuse. Benzodiazepines may also be useful for acute symptoms during the period before an SSRI takes effect or as an adjunct for partial responders to SSRIs or SNRIs.[50]

Delirium

Delirium is among the most common neuropsychiatric syndromes encountered in patients with advanced medical illness. It is relevant because it is associated with increased rates of morbidity and mortality.[51] There are many causes and conditions that lead to the constellation of symptoms observed. Several potential causes are often present at the same time. It has been reported that delirium may be reversible in up to 50% of cases.[52] This finding is of particular importance when clinicians consider its cause and how to treat it.

The presentation of delirium can be variable, although patients typically present with some change in cognition and attention.

The American Psychiatric Association's Diagnostic and Statistical Manual, Fifth edition, describes 5 characteristics of delirium[48]:

- Disturbance in attention (reduced ability to direct, focus, sustain, shift attention) and awareness.
- The disturbance develops over a short period of time (usually hours to days), represents a change from baseline, and tends to fluctuate during the course of the day.
- An additional disturbance in cognition (memory deficit, disorientation, language, visuospatial ability, or perception).
- The disturbances are not better explained by another preexisting, evolving, or established neurocognitive disorder, and do not occur in the context of a severely reduced level of arousal, such as coma.
- There is evidence from the history, physical examination, or laboratory findings that the disturbance is caused by a medical condition, substance intoxication, or withdrawal, or medication side effect.

Some of the most frequent causes of delirium in oncology patients are[53]:

- Infection
- Metabolic derangements (increased calcium level, decreased sodium level, renal failure)
- Central nervous system primary or metastatic disease/edema
- Medication related (eg, opioids, psychotropics, steroids)

- Cancer treatment (chemotherapy, radiation therapy)
- Sleep deprivation
- Paraneoplastic neurologic syndromes

Optimizing Pharmacologic Management

As with all symptoms discussed here, the underlying cause must first be treated. If a person's delirium is related to a new infection, the appropriate antibiotics will suffice. Because many medications may also provoke delirium (opioids and other psychoactive medications) it is important to review medication lists and limit offensive agents. In cases of refractory or terminal delirium, neuroleptics are the first-line treatment. Benzodiazepines should be avoided unless the source of delirium is alcohol-sedative drug withdrawal because they can be associated with paradoxic worsening of confusion.

Haloperidol is the neuroleptic agent of choice for most patients. It has a limited side effect profile and can be administered safely through oral and parenteral routes. Older-generation neuroleptics are able to control symptoms but they may have a higher incidence of side effects: extrapyramidal reactions, sedation, and hypotension (ie, Thorazine). New-generation neuroleptics such as olanzapine, quetiapine, and risperidone are also used in the management of confusional states and show fewer side effects; however they are limited in their supporting evidence and ability to be given parenterally.

Noninvasive Management

Supportive measures that rely on a nonpharmacologic approach can be successful and should be used. Patients who have recovered from delirium have reported that simple communication, reality orientation, a visible clock, and presence of a relative are all helpful factors that contribute to heightened sense of control during the episode.[54,55]

Other strategies to consider using:

- Establish a quiet environment: limiting excess noise and stimulation by staff and visitors
- Ensure patients have glasses, hearing aids, dentures
- Have objects from the patient's home environment present (eg, pictures, blankets, sleepwear)
- Provide adequate lighting
- Make available clear, visible signs providing the patient's location and date

SUMMARY

Symptom management is an undertaking that, at its best, uses an interdisciplinary approach. To best support individuals living with a cancer diagnosis, it is imperative to mobilize the collective skills and expertise of the entire medical/psychosocial team. If available as a resource, early palliative-care support has been shown to improve the outcomes of patients with cancer, even if mobilized in late disease. If a palliative-care team is not available, then there are many resources for clinicians to consult in order to provide the best possible care for their patients.

Any symptom that manifests can be prevented or managed, regardless of when it occurs or to what it is related. Whether symptoms manifest at the time of diagnosis, during treatment, or years after a cure has been established, clinicians must remain vigilant in their understanding and approach to supporting patients' suffering. Developing a common approach to interviewing patients, assessing concerns, and recommending a treatment plan can benefit both the consistency of a practice, and the symptom burden of the patients. In this common approach, clinicians must be aware of special circumstances that may influence their diagnostic and treatment strategy. With these skills, advanced practice clinicians can help to extend the ideals and practice of palliative care to improve the quality of life of their patients and diminish their suffering at end of life.

REFERENCES

1. Field MJ, Cassel CK, editors. Approaching death: improving care at the end of life. Washington, DC: National Academy Press; 1997.
2. A controlled trial to improve care for seriously ill hospitalized patients. The Study to Understand Prognoses and Preferences for Outcomes and Risks of Treatments (SUPPORT). The SUPPORT Principal Investigators. JAMA 1995;274:1591–8.
3. Manfredi PI, Morrison RS, Morris J, et al. Palliative care consultations: how do they impact the care of hospitalized patients? J Pain Symptom Manage 2000; 20:166–73.
4. Williams M, Wheeler M. Palliative care: what is it? Home Healthc Nurse 2001; 19(9):550–6.
5. Temel J, Greer JA, Muzikansky A, et al. Early palliative care for patients with met-astatic non-small-cell lung cancer. N Engl J Med 2010;363:733–42.
6. Billings A. What is palliative care? J Palliat Care 1998;1:73–81.
7. Morrison S. Palliative care. N Engl J Med 2004;350:2582–90.
8. Meffert C, Gaertner J, Seibel K, et al. Early palliative care–health services research and implementation of sustainable changes: the study protocol of the EVI project. BMC Cancer 2015;15:443.
9. Available at: https://reportcard.capc.org/. Accessed November 23, 2015.
10. Available at: https://www.capc.org/. Accessed November 23, 2015.
11. Pollak AN, Gulli B, Chatelain L, et al. Emergency care and transportation of the sick and injured. 9th edition. Sudbury (MA): Jones and Bartlett; 2005. p. 148–9.
12. Homsi J, Walsh D, Rivera N, et al. Symptom evaluation in palliative medicine: pa-tient report vs systematic assessment. Support Care Cancer 2006;14:444.
13. Dudel J. General sensory physiology, psychophysics. In: Dude J, editor. Funda-mentals of sensory physiology, general sensory physiology, psychophysics. New York: Springer Verlag; 1977. p. 1.
14. Schwartz AL, Meek PM, Nail LM, et al. Measurement of fatigue. determining mini-mally important clinical differences. J Clin Epidemiol 2002;55:239.
15. Symptom assessment and management tools. Available at: https://www.cancercare.on.ca/toolbox/symptools/. Accessed September 10, 2014.
16. Tranmer JE, Heyland D, Dudgeon D, et al. Measuring the symptom experience of seriously ill cancer and noncancer hospitalized patients near the end of life with the memorial symptom assessment scale. J Pain Symptom Manage 2003;25:420.
17. Cleeland CS, Mendoza TR, Wang XS, et al. Assessing symptom distress in can-cer patients: the M.D. Anderson Symptom Inventory. Cancer 2000;89:1634.
18. de Haes JC, van Knippenberg FC, Neijt JP. Measuring psychological and phys-ical distress in cancer patients: structure and application of the Rotterdam Symp-tom Checklist. Br J Cancer 1990;62:1034.
19. McCorkle R. The measurement of symptom distress. Semin Oncol Nurs 1987;3:248.
20. The National Comprehensive Cancer Network Distress Thermometer. Available at: http://www.nccn.org/patients/resources/life_with_cancer/distress.aspx. Ac-cessed November 17, 2015.

21. Miaskowski C, Leary J, Burney R, et al. Guideline for the management of cancer pain in adults and children, APS clinical practice guidelines series, No. 3. Glenview (IL): American Pain Society; 2005.
22. Available at: http://www.who.int/cancer/palliative/painladder/en/. Accessed December 9, 2015.
23. Abrahm JA. A physician's guide to pain and symptom management in cancer patients. Baltimore (MD): Johns Hopkins University Press.; 2005.
24. Abrahm J. Physician's guide to pain and symptom management in cancer patients. Baltimore (MD): The Johns Hopkins University Press; 2014. p. 460–4.
25. Cancer.gov. Education in palliative care for oncology: self study module 3m: symptoms, Malignant pleural effusions. Available at: http://www.cancer.gov/resources-for/hp/education/epeco/self-study/module-3/module-3m.pdf. Accessed December 17, 2015.
26. Cancer.gov. Education in palliative care for oncology: self study module 3j: dyspnea. Available at: http://www.cancer.gov/resources-for/hp/education/epeco/self-study/module-3/module-3j.pdf. Accessed December 17, 2015.
27. Sabriski L. Interventional approaches to oncological pain management. In: Berger A, Portenoy RK, Weissman DE, editors. Principles and practice of supportive oncology. Philadelphia: Lippincott-Raven Publishers; 1998.
28. Karkauer E. Case records of the Massachusetts General Hospital. Weekly clinico-pathological exercises. Case 6-2005. A 58-year-old man with esophageal cancer and nausea, vomiting, and intractable hiccups. N Engl J Med 2005;352(8):817–25.
29. Abrahm J. Physician's guide to pain and symptom management in cancer patients. Baltimore (MD): The Johns Hopkins University Press; 2014. p. 450–60.
30. Available at: http://www.cancer.gov/about-cancer/treatment/side-effects/constipation/GI-complications-hp-pdq#section/_8. Accessed December 28, 2015.
31. Badke, A. Fast Facts #294 Opioid induced constipation part 1: established management strategies. Available at: https://www.capc.org/fast-facts/294-opiod-induced-constipation-part-1-established-management-strategies/. Accessed December 28, 2015.
32. Abrahm J. Physician's guide to pain and symptom management in cancer patients. Baltimore (MD): The Johns Hopkins University Press; 2014. p. 238.
33. Alderman, J. Fast Fact #96. Diarrhea in palliative care. Available at: https://www.capc.org/fast-facts/96-diarrhea-palliative-care/. Accessed December 28, 2015.
34. Abrahm J. Physician's guide to pain and symptom management in cancer patients. Baltimore (MD): The Johns Hopkins University Press; 2014. p. 449.
35. Available at: http://www.cancer.gov/about-cancer/treatment/side-effects/constipation/GI-complications-hp-pdq#section/_119. Accessed December 28, 2015.
36. Reisfield GM, Wilson GR. Fast Fact #173 Cancer related fatigue. Available at: https://www.capc.org/fast-facts/173-cancer-related-fatigue/. Accessed December 28, 2015.
37. Sarhill N. Methylphenidate for fatigue in advanced cancer: a prospective open-label pilot study. Am J Hosp Palliat Care 2001;18:187–92.
38. Rozans M. Palliative uses of methylphenidate in patients with cancer: a review. J Clin Oncol 2002;20:335–9.
39. Ahlberg K, Ekman T, Gaston-Johansson F, et al. Assessment and management of cancer-related fatigue. Lancet 2003;362(9384):640–50.
40. Mock V. Evidence-based treatment of cancer-related fatigue. J Natl Cancer Inst Monogr 2004;(32):112–8.
41. Ferris F. Fast Fact #37 Pruritus. Available at: https://www.capc.org/fast-facts/37-pruritus/. Accessed December 28, 2015.

42. Cancer.gov. Dealing with side effects. Available at: http://www.cancer.gov/about-cancer/treatment/side-effects/skin-nail-changes/pruritus-pdq#section/_23. Accessed November 20, 2015.

43. Maione P, Perrone F, Gallo C, et al. Pretreatment quality of life and functional status assessment significantly predict survival of elderly patients with advanced non-small-cell lung cancer receiving chemotherapy: a prognostic analysis of the Multicenter Italian Lung Cancer in the Elderly Study. J Clin Oncol 2005;23: 6865–72.

44. Movsas B, Moughan J, Sarna L, et al. Quality of life supersedes the classic prognosticators for long-term survival in locally advanced non-small-cell lung cancer: an analysis of RTOG 9801. J Clin Oncol 2009;27:5816–22.

45. Pirl WF, Temel JS, Billings A, et al. Depression after diagnosis of advanced non-small cell lung cancer and survival: a pilot study. Psychosomatics 2008;49: 218–24.

46. Mitchell AJ, Chan M, Bhatti H, et al. Prevalence of depression, anxiety, and adjustment disorder in oncological, haematological, and palliative-care settings: a meta-analysis of 94 interview-based studies. Lancet Oncol 2011;12:160–74.

47. Boyes A, Girgis A, D'Este CA, et al. Prevalence and predictors of the short-term trajectory of anxiety and depression in the first year after a cancer diagnosis: a population based longitudinal study. J Clin Oncol 2013;44:7540.

48. Diagnostic and statistical manual of mental disorders – fifth edition. Washington, DC: American Psychiatric Association, APA Press; 2013.

49. von Wolff A, Hölzel LP, Westphal A, et al. Selective serotonin reuptake inhibitors and tricyclic antidepressants in the acute treatment of chronic depression and dysthymia: a systematic review and meta-analysis. J Affect Disord 2013;144:7.

50. Kapczinski F, Lima MS, Souza JS, et al. Antidepressants for generalized anxiety disorder. Cochrane Database Syst Rev 2003;(2):CD003592.

51. Levkoff SE, Evans DA, Liptzin B, et al. Delirium: the occurrence and persistence of symptoms among elderly hospitalized patients. Arch Intern Med 1992;152: 334–40.

52. Casarett DJ, Inouye SK, American College of Physicians–American Society of Internal Medicine End-of-Life Care Consensus Panel. Diagnosis and management of delirium near the end of life. Ann Intern Med 2001;135:32.

53. Bruera E, Neumann CM. Management of specific symptom complexes in patients receiving palliative care. CMAJ 1998;158:1717.

54. Inouye SK, Bogardus ST, Williams CS, et al. The role of adherence on the effectiveness of nonpharmacologic interventions: evidence from the delirium prevention trial. Arch Intern Med 2003;163:958–64.

55. Blinderman C, Billings JA. Comfort care for patients dying in the hospital. N Engl J Med 2015;373:2549–61.

Oncologic Emergencies

Katherine L. Kunstel, MMSc, PA-C[a,b,c],*

KEYWORDS

- Febrile neutropenia • Hypercalcemia • Tumor lysis syndrome • Cancer emergencies

KEY POINTS

- Febrile neutropenia warrants appropriate microbiology cultures, imaging, and prompt administration of empiric broad-spectrum antibiotics. Fever may be the only indication of infection in a neutropenic patient.
- Patients with hypercalcemia of malignancy present with a range of symptoms. Aggressive intravenous hydration and administration of bisphosphonates is the cornerstone of treatment for patients with hypercalcemia of malignancy.
- Tumor lysis syndrome occurs when an influx of uric acid, potassium, and phosphorus overwhelms the body's homeostatic mechanisms. Identification of at-risk patients and prevention with aggressive hydration and allopurinol are key.

INTRODUCTION

People who have cancer, and those who are being treated for cancer, represent a patient population with risk factors for certain life-threatening conditions, which are referred to as *oncologic emergencies*. Many conditions are considered oncologic emergencies but some that are common include febrile neutropenia (FN), hypercalcemia of malignancy, and tumor lysis syndrome (TLS). Clinicians who practice in oncology are accustomed to managing these acute conditions; however, given that many patients present to their primary care physician, emergency room, or urgent care center when they become ill, it is prudent that clinicians outside of oncology are familiar with common oncologic emergencies. Knowledge of risk factors, recognition of presenting features, diagnostic workup, and appropriate intervention are essential to provide the best care for patients with oncologic emergencies.

FEBRILE NEUTROPENIA

FN is a common complication of chemotherapy for people with cancer. FN is particularly concerning for patients treated for hematologic malignancies, given the

Disclosure Statement: The author has nothing to disclose.
[a] Department of Physician Assistant Studies, College of Health Professions, Lenox Hill Hospital, Pace University, 163 William Street, Fifth Floor, New York, NY 10038, USA; [b] Smilow Cancer Hospital, Yale-New Haven Hospital, 20 York Street, New Haven, CT 06510, USA; [c] New York-Presbyterian Hospital, 630 West 168th Street, New York, NY 10032, USA
* Department of Physician Assistant Studies, Pace University-Lenox Hill Hospital, 163 William Street, Fifth Floor, New York, NY 10038.
E-mail address: kkunstel@pace.edu

Physician Assist Clin 1 (2016) 397–408
http://dx.doi.org/10.1016/j.cpha.2016.03.002
2405-7991/16/$ – see front matter © 2016 Elsevier Inc. All rights reserved.
physicianassistant.theclinics.com

myelosuppressive nature of those chemotherapy regimens. FN is deemed an oncologic emergency because infections can progress rapidly in these patients; therefore, immediate medical attention is warranted.

NEUTROPENIA

Neutropenia is defined by the absolute neutrophil count (ANC). ANC is the sum of circulating segmented and band neutrophils. Neutropenia is further characterized in terms of severity. Although there is some variability, typically an ANC less than 1.0×10^9/L is considered neutropenia. Severe neutropenia is an ANC less than 0.5×10^9/L or an ANC that is expected to decrease to less than this level within 48 hours, and profound neutropenia refers to an ANC less than 0.1×10^9/L.[1] As the severity and duration of neutropenia increases, so does the risk of infection.

FEVER

The Infectious Diseases Society of America defines fever in neutropenic patients as a single temperature measurement by oral or tympanic membrane of $\geq38.3°C$ (101°F) or a temperature of greater than 38°C (100.4°F) for greater than one hour.[1]

DIAGNOSIS

Febrile neutropenia is considered a medical emergency and calls for immediate evaluation and intervention by a medical professional. All patients should have a detailed history taken and physical examination performed. Time is of the essence, as these patients may quickly become hemodynamically unstable. Fever may be the only presenting sign of infection in neutropenic patients, as they may not be able to mount a typical inflammatory response. Signs of infection may be absent or subtle. For example, skin and soft tissue infections may not have associated erythema or induration. In addition, patients with neutropenia are unlikely to be able to form an abscess.

A history should include a complete review of systems, use of any prophylactic antimicrobial agents, recent use of therapeutic antimicrobial agents, previous infections, and comorbidities. Physical examination should be thorough and include sites most likely to be infected and any site identified as being of concern while taking the patient's history. Common sites of infection include the skin, catheter insertion sites, the oral mucosa, sinuses, lungs, abdomen, genitals, and perianal areas. It is imperative to avoid digital rectal examination in these patients, as infection can be introduced by the manipulation of the fragile mucosa of the anus.[1]

Laboratory evaluation should include a complete blood count with differential, comprehensive metabolic panel, coagulation panel, and urinalysis. Microbiology evaluation should include blood and urine cultures. At minimum, 2 sets of blood cultures should be drawn from each patient. If the patient has an indwelling catheter, one set of blood cultures should be drawn from each lumen of the patient's catheter and from the periphery.[1] Pursuing diagnostic imaging tends to be institution dependent. Chest radiographs may be obtained or computed tomography of the chest may be warranted depending on reported respiratory symptoms or signs on physical examination. Abdominal imaging is not typically performed unless some aspect of the patient's history or physical examination suggests an abdominal source of infection.

Only some cases of FN will have an infectious agent identified. Historically, gram-negative organisms were most commonly isolated; however, that has now shifted to gram-positive organisms. This shift is thought to be related to several practice changes, including use of long-term indwelling central venous catheters (CVCs),[2] empiric antibiotic regimens targeting *Pseudomonas aeruginosa*, antimicrobial prophylaxis, and new chemotherapy regimens.

MANAGEMENT

Empiric broad-spectrum antibiotics should be administered within 1 hour of fever documentation.[1,3,4] Dose adjustments should be made accordingly for any hepatic or kidney dysfunction.[1,5] Antibiotic therapy should cover both gram-positive and gram-negative organisms, ensuring coverage for *P aeruginosa*. The Infectious Diseases Society of America recommends empiric monotherapy with an antipseudomonal β-lactam agent, such as cefepime (2 g intravenously [IV] every 8 hours), ceftazidime (2 g IV every 8 hours), imipenem-cilastatin (500 mg IV every 6 hours), meropenem (1 g IV every 8 hours), or piperacillin-tazobactam (4.5 g IV every 6 hours).[1,3] Note that the dose administration when treating patients with FN varies from standard dosing (**Table 1**). Vancomycin is not recommended to be used as part of fist-line therapy but can be added for skin and soft tissue infections, severe mucositis, sepsis or hemodynamic instability, pneumonia, or if an indwelling line is suspected as a source of infection.[1]

The initial antimicrobial regimen should be continued until defervescence and then for a minimum of 2 to 3 days afterwards.[6] If Vancomycin or other specific gram-positive coverage was started empirically, it can be discontinued after 48 hours if there is no evidence of gram-positive infection.[1,5] If a causative organism is identified, then antibiotics should be continued at minimum for the standard treatment of that infection and until the ANC recovers to more than 500. If fever persists without a causative organism identified, then empiric antifungal coverage should be added after 5 to 7 days of broad-spectrum, empiric antibiotics.

INDWELLING CATHETERS

It is important to document the time peripheral and central blood cultures were drawn. If blood cultures that are drawn from CVC become positive at least 2 hours prior to when peripherally drawn blood cultures become positive, then it is likely that the CVC is the source of infection.[1] The Infectious Diseases Society of America recommends removal of the CVC if the following organisms are identified as the cause of infection: *Staphylococcus aureus*, *P aeruginosa*, *Candida* species, and mycobacteria. Other indications for removal of the CVC are sepsis with hemodynamic compromise, persistent bacteremia after 72 hours in spite of appropriate antibiotic coverage, and tunnel infection.[6] It is recommended to continue antibiotics for at least 14 days after removal of the CVC and clearance of blood cultures.[1,3,4]

Table 1	
Empiric antibiotic monotherapy agents and dosing for febrile neutropenia	
Antibiotic	**Dose**
Cefepime	2 g IV every 8 h
Ceftazidime	2 g IV every 8 h
Imipenem-cilastatin	500 mg IV every 6 h
Meropenem	1 g IV every 8 h
Piperacillin-tazobactam	4.5 g IV every 6 h

For patients with normal renal function.

HYPERCALCEMIA OF MALIGNANCY

Hypercalcemia of malignancy occurs in up to 30% of patients with cancer at some point during the course of their disease.[7] Hypercalcemia is more likely to occur in patients with an established cancer diagnosis and those with advanced disease. Among those hospitalized with hypercalcemia, malignancy is the most common cause.[8] Breast cancer, lung cancer, renal cell carcinomas, multiple myeloma, and T-cell leukemia/lymphoma are most often implicated in hypercalcemia.[9,10]

PATHOPHYSIOLOGY

Several mechanisms drive hypercalcemia in malignancy. Most commonly, hypercalcemia is caused by the production of parathyroid hormone–related protein (PTHrP) by the tumor itself.[11] PTHrP is structurally similar to parathyroid hormone and can mimic its effects on the bone and kidney, leading to increased bone resorption and calcium reabsorption in the distal tubule, respectively. Bone metastases may stimulate factors such as cytokines that stimulate osteoclasts, leading to bone destruction and hypercalcemia.[12,13] Less commonly, hypercalcemia may result from the overproduction of vitamin D analogues, such as calcitriol.[14] This is more often seen in hematologic malignancies.

DIAGNOSIS

Generally, patients with hypercalcemia present with vague complaints such as lethargy, confusion, nausea, constipation, polyuria, or polydipsia. Hypercalcemia may also be found incidentally as a laboratory abnormality.[12] The presence and severity of symptoms tends to depend on how rapidly the calcium level increases. As with many things, the body is more able to adapt if the increase in calcium is gradual over an extended period than if it increases acutely.[15]

Ionized serum calcium should be used to make the diagnosis and to monitor for response to treatment. If total serum calcium is used, it must be corrected for the serum albumin level. Corrected calcium = total calcium + (0.8 × [4.0-albumin]). Serum creatinine should be monitored as well as electrolytes. The measurement of PTHrP has not been proven to affect outcomes and should not guide initial management, but it can add prognostic information. Patients with elevated PTHrP levels (>12 pmol/L) have been found to be less responsive to bisphosphonate therapy and more prone to develop recurrent hypercalcemia.[16]

MANAGEMENT

Recognition of symptomatic hypercalcemia and urgent intervention is paramount. IV hydration with normal saline is the cornerstone of management, as almost all patients with hypercalcemia present with intravascular volume depletion. Intravenous fluids should be administered aggressively (500–1000 mL in the first hour and then continuously at 150–250 mL/h) to restore intravascular volume and achieve brisk urine output.[17] Consideration must be given to the patient's cardiac and pulmonary status in relation to IV fluid administration. Once the patient is euvolemic, loop diuretics, such as furosemide, can be added to promote calciuresis. Medications that act to increase the calcium level, such as vitamin D and thiazide diuretics, should be avoided. Intravenous phosphates should also be avoided, as they can potentially cause calciphylaxis—calcification and necrosis of the skin and adipose tissue—especially when the calcium-phosphate product exceeds 70 mg/dL.[18]

In addition to IV fluids, bisphosphonates (zoledronic acid and pamidronate) can be used to decrease calcium levels. Bisphosphonates work by inhibiting osteoclastic bone resorption, and are considered a mainstay of treatment for hypercalcemia of malignancy. The onset of action of bisphosphonates is 24 to 72 hours, and calcium levels reach their lowest point about 1 week after administration. Common adverse effects include bone pain, ocular inflammation,[19] electrolyte abnormalities including "overshoot" hypocalcemia,[20] and atrial dysrhythmias.[21] Less commonly, osteonecrosis of the jaw can occur in those patients with poor dentition. Both zoledronic acid and pamidronate are cleared renally and must be used with caution in those with renal impairment. Hemodialysis may be a safer and more efficient way of correcting hypercalcemia in those with kidney dysfunction.[22] Hemodialysis may also be the route of management in those with congestive heart failure or other conditions that limit the administration of aggressive IV fluids.[23]

Given the slower onset of action of bisphosphonates, subcutaneous or intramuscular calcitonin can be given in conjunction with IV fluid administration to lower calcium levels more quickly. Nasal administration is not effective in this setting.[24,25] Calcitonin should not be used for longer than 72 hours and should not be used as a single agent in the treatment of hypercalcemia because of the associated increased risk of tachyphylaxis and rebound hypercalcemia.

Steroids can also be used in limited duration for those patients who have persistent hypercalcemia in spite of bisphosphonate administration.[26] Glucocorticoids help with mediating the release of cytokines and prostaglandins that stimulate osteoclasts and also inhibit calcitriol production by macrophages.[18] Toxicities associated with glucocorticoids limit their use (**Fig. 1**).

TUMOR LYSIS SYNDROME

TLS is a potentially life-threatening emergency that is characterized by metabolic abnormalities that occur when tumor cells release their intracellular contents into the circulation and overwhelm the body's homeostatic mechanisms. TLS commonly occurs in the setting of bulky tumors, rapidly proliferating tumors, and tumors that are responsive to therapy, most commonly in hematologic malignancies such as acute lymphoblastic leukemia and Burkitt's lymphoma, but can also occur with solid tumors. TLS can arise spontaneously but more often develops after initiation of therapy.

PATHOPHYSIOLOGY

When tumor cells lyse, electrolytes, proteins, and nucleic acids are released into the bloodstream. This sudden influx can result in hyperuricemia, hyperkalemia, and hyperphosphatemia with subsequent hypocalcemia and have potentially detrimental effects on the kidneys, myocardium, and central nervous system.

The release and catabolism of nucleic acids, specifically purine nucleic acids that are metabolized by xanthine oxidase into uric acid, can lead to hyperuricemia. In this environment, crystal formation and deposition increase, which may lead to renal insufficiency or failure.[27,28]

It is estimated that the level of phosphorus in cancer cells may be up to 4 times the levels found in normal cells; thus, the rapid release of this intracellular phosphorus can lead to hyperphosphatemia.[27] The kidneys initially act to remedy this by increasing excretion and decreasing tubular resorption; however, the kidneys can become overwhelmed. Acute kidney injury caused by uricemia may further exacerbate the

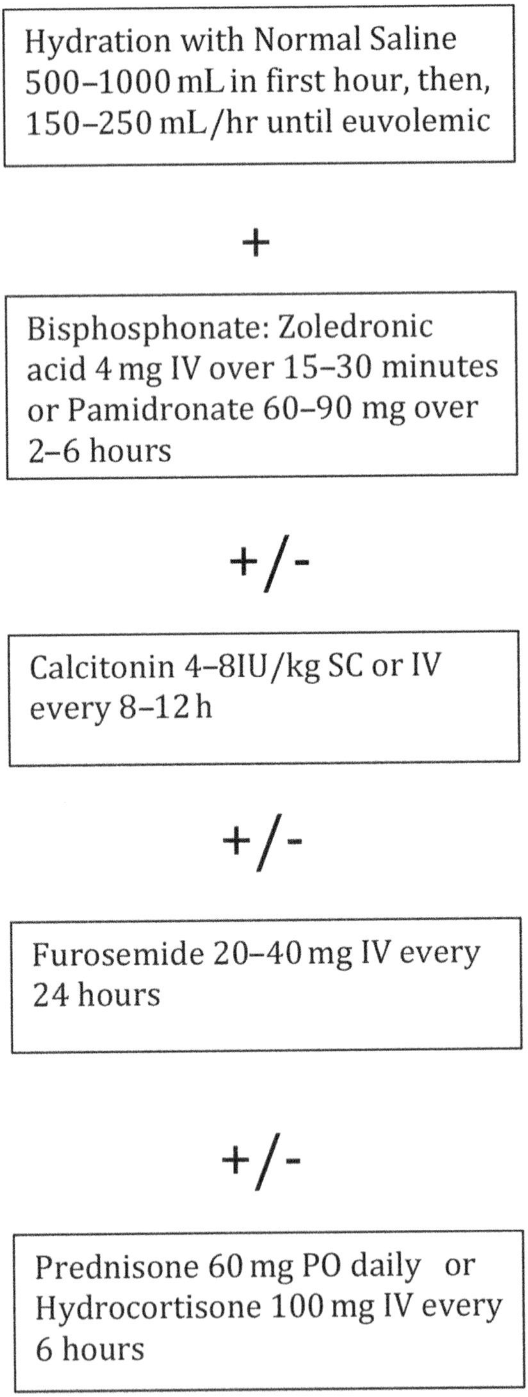

Hydration with Normal Saline
500–1000 mL in first hour, then,
150–250 mL/hr until euvolemic

+

Bisphosphonate: Zoledronic
acid 4 mg IV over 15–30 minutes
or Pamidronate 60–90 mg over
2–6 hours

+/−

Calcitonin 4–8IU/kg SC or IV
every 8–12 h

+/−

Furosemide 20–40 mg IV every
24 hours

+/−

Prednisone 60 mg PO daily or
Hydrocortisone 100 mg IV every
6 hours

Fig. 1. Treatment of hypercalcemia of malignancy. PO, oral; SC, subcutaneous; IV, intravenous.

development of hyperphosphatemia.[29] Furthermore, there is an increased likelihood of calcium phosphate precipitation when the calcium-phosphorus product exceeds 70,[27,30,31] thereby increasing the precipitation of calcium phosphate in the renal tubules and further exacerbating renal injury.[32]

Hypocalcemia is a consequence of hyperphosphatemia and is included in the metabolic derangements that constitute TLS.

Hyperkalemia results from the rapid release of intracellular potassium into the bloodstream. This may be worsened by renal failure in the setting of TLS. Hyperkalemia may provoke cardiac irregularities ranging from arrhythmias to cardiac arrest.[33]

CLINICAL PRESENTATION AND DIAGNOSIS

TLS can be diagnosed based on both laboratory and clinical findings. To help make the diagnosis, the definitions of clinical TLS and laboratory TLS were standardized by Cairo and Bishop in 2004. Based on their classification, laboratory TLS occurs when 2 or more metabolic values are abnormal or if they change by 25% within 3 days before or 7 days after initiation of therapy (**Table 2**).[34–38] Clinical TLS is defined as the presence of laboratory TLS with the addition of one of the following clinically relevant complications: renal insufficiency, cardiac arrhythmias, seizures, and sudden death (**Table 3**).[38]

Patients with TLS may present with a range of symptoms. Acute obstructive uropathy can cause hematuria, flank pain, hypertension, azotemia, acidosis, edema, oliguria, anuria, lethargy, and somnolence.[36]

Hyperkalemia can cause gastrointestinal distress, such as nausea, vomiting, diarrhea, and anorexia. High serum potassium levels can also provoke muscle weakness, cramps, and paresthesias. The most serious manifestations of hyperkalemia, as noted earlier, are the cardiac abnormalities (peaked T waves or widened QRS on electrocardiogram [ECG], arrhythmias, asystole, syncope) and risk of sudden death.[36,37]

Patients with severe hyperphosphatemia may experience nausea, vomiting, diarrhea, lethargy, and seizures. Meanwhile, severe hypocalcemia is associated with muscular effects (muscle cramps, paresthesias, tetany), cardiac abnormalities (arrhythmias, heart block, hypotension), and neurologic consequences (confusion, delirium, seizures).

MANAGEMENT

Prevention is key in the management of TLS. Therefore, identification of those at risk for TLS and being proactive with intervention is paramount. Aggressive IV hydration is a cornerstone of supportive care along with vigilant electrolyte monitoring before and during treatment. Hydration should be initiated at least 24 hours before cytoreductive therapy. Intravenous hydration promotes increased urine flow, which results in improved intravascular volume, renal perfusion, and glomerular filtration, all of which promote excretion of uric acid and phosphate.[39–41] Loop diuretics may also be used to

Table 2		
Cairo-Bishop definition of laboratory TLS		
Metabolites	**Value**	**Change from Baseline**
Uric acid	≥476 µmol/L or 8 mg/dL	25% increase
Potassium	≥6 mEq/L or 6 mg/dL	25% increase
Phosphorus	≥2.1 mmol/L (children) ≥1.45 mmol/L (adults)	25% increase
Calcium	≤1.75 mmol/L	25% decrease

Adapted from Cairo M, Bishop M. Tumor lysis syndrome: new therapeutic strategies and classification. Br J Haematol 2004;127:5; with permission.

Table 3
Cairo-Bishop TLS definition and grading of clinical TLS

Complication	0	1	2	3	4	5
				Grade		
Creatinine	≤1.5 × ULN	1.5 × ULN	>1.5–3.0 × ULN	>3.0–6.0 × ULN	>6.0 × ULN	Death
Cardiac arrhythmia	None	Intervention not indicated	Nonurgent medical intervention indicated	Symptomatic and incompletely controlled with device (eg, defibrillator)	Life threatening (eg, arrhythmia associated with CHF, hypotension, syncope, shock)	Death
Seizure	None	—	One brief generalized seizure; seizures well controlled by anticonvulsants or infrequent focal motor seizures not interfering with ADL	Seizure in which consciousness is altered; poorly controlled seizure disorder; with breakthrough generalized seizure despite intervention	Seizures of any kind that are prolonged, repetitive, or difficult to control (eg, status epilepticus, intractable epilepsy)	Death

Abbreviations: ADL, activities of daily living; CHF, congestive heart failure; ULN, upper limit of normal.
From Cairo M, Bishop M. Tumor lysis syndrome: new therapeutic strategies and classification. Br J Haematol 2004;127:6; with permission.

maintain brisk urine flow; however, they are contraindicated in patients with hypovolemia or obstructive uropathy. In the past, the use of sodium bicarbonate for urine alkalinization was a standard practice for the prevention and treatment of TLS; however, there is lack of evidence showing its efficacy, and urinary alkalinization is no longer recommended.[37]

The standard of care for hyperuricemia is aggressive hydration and the use of a hypouricemic agent, such as allopurinol or rasburicase. Allopurinol is a xanthine analogue, which when converted in vivo to oxypurinol, is a competitive inhibitor of xanthine oxidase and thereby blocks the conversion of xanthine and hypoxanthine to uric acid.[42,43] Allopurinol is found to decrease the formation of uric acid and reduce the incidence of obstructive uropathy in patients who are at risk for TLS.[42] Allopurinol should be used as prophylaxis, initiated 1 to 2 days before cytoreductive therapy, and continued for 3 to 7 days depending on the ongoing risk assessment for TLS.[17] The recommended dose for allopurinol in this setting is 100 mg/m^2 per dose every 8 hours (maximum, 800 mg/d) orally or 200 to 400 mg/m^2/d in 1 to 3 divided doses IV (max 600 mg/d).[37] Side effects include gastrointestinal upset, rash, fever, xanthine nephrolithiasis, and allergic reactions. Allopurinol is renally excreted, so dose adjustments need to be made in patients with renal insufficiency.[44] Note that allopurinol has a slow onset of action and has no effect in the excretion of uric acid that has already formed, thereby reinforcing its role as a prophylactic agent.

Rasburicase is a recombinant urate oxidase that converts uric acid into water-soluble allantoin. It has been approved by the US Food and Drug Administration for use as the initial management of hyperuricemia in pediatric and adult patients undergoing therapy for leukemia, lymphoma, or solid tumors who are at risk of TLS and subsequent hyperuricemia. The approved dose is 0.2 mg/kg infused over 30 minutes daily for up to 5 days.[17] However, rasburicase is found to be effective in lowering uric acid levels after only 1 dose. Therefore, clinicians generally give a 1-time fixed dose of 3, 6, or 7.5 mg or a weight-based dose of either 0.05 or 0.15 mg/kg.[17] Side effects of rasburicase can include minor allergic reactions, headaches, itching, edema, wheezing, and anaphylaxis. Rasburicase is contraindicated for use in pregnant and lactating women and in those with glucose-6-phosphate dehydrogenase deficiency (**Table 4**).[45]

Table 4		
Treatment of TLS: antihyperuricemic agents		
Agent	**Mechanism of Action**	**Recommendations**
Allopurinol	Inhibits xanthine oxidase, which converts hypoxanthine and xanthine to uric acid in the purine catabolism pathway	• Dosing: 100 mg/m^2/dose every 8 h PO (maximum, 800 mg/d) or 200–400 mg/m^2/d in 1–3 divided doses IV (maximum, 600 mg/d) • Reduce dose by 50% in renal failure • 6-mercaptopurine and/or azathioprine doses must be reduced when given concomitantly with allopurinol
Rasburicase	Converts uric acid to highly soluble allantoin in the purine catabolism pathway	• Administration: infuse IV over 30 min; dose is based on risk assessment of TLS and baseline uric acid levels • Contraindicated in G6PD deficiency patients and those with a known history of reaction to rasburicase • Uric acid levels should be monitored regularly and used as a guide to modulate dosing

Abbreviations: G6PD, glucose-6-phosphate dehydrogenase; PO, orally.
Data from Cairo M, Bishop M. Tumor lysis syndrome: new therapeutic strategies and classification. Br J Haematol 2004;127:8.

Hyperkalemia usually occurs 6 to 72 hours after cytoreductive therapy is initiated and can intensify in the setting of acute kidney injury.[46] Serum potassium may be acutely reduced by several mechanisms including administration of 10 U of regular insulin, immediately followed by 50 mL of 50% dextrose, and then an hour-long infusion of 50 to 75 mL 10% dextrose to prevent hypoglycemia[47]; inhaled β-agonists (eg, 20 mg of nebulized albuterol)[48]; and use of loop diuretics. Sodium bicarbonate and a slow infusion of calcium gluconate with ECG monitoring can be used to treat life-threatening arrhythmias.[17] In some cases, hemodialysis is necessary.

Hyperphosphatemia usually occurs 24 to 48 hours after induction of cytotoxic therapy, and is managed with a low phosphorus diet and short-term use of oral phosphate binders like aluminum hydroxide (300 mg with meals) or aluminum carbonate (30 mL every 6 hours). Calcium carbonate should be avoided in patients with hypercalcemia.

Asymptomatic hypocalcemia is not routinely treated in patients with TLS because of the risk of precipitation in the setting of hyperphosphatemia. Hypocalcemia generally improves without intervention as the TLS resolves. In patients who have symptomatic hypocalcemia, slow IV administration of calcium gluconate can be given with ECG monitoring.[17]

SUMMARY/DISCUSSION

Oncologic emergencies are common, potentially life-threatening conditions that affect people with cancer and those being treated for cancer. Clinicians should be aware of the risk factors, presenting features, diagnostic workup, and appropriate intervention for these acute conditions. This review was limited to febrile neutropenia, hypercalcemia, and tumor lysis syndrome; however, there are many other conditions considered to warrant emergent intervention in people who have cancer. Familiarity with common oncologic emergencies will lead to better care and likely to better outcomes for these at-risk patients.

REFERENCES

1. Freifield AG, Bow EJ, Sepkowitz KA, et al. Clinical practice guideline for the use of antimicrobial agents in neutropenic patients with cancer: 2010 update by the Infectious Diseases Society of America. Clin Infect Dis 2011;52: e56–93.
2. Raad I, Chaftari AM. Advances in prevention and management of central-line associated bloodstream infections in patients with cancer. Clin Infect Dis 2014; 59(Suppl 5):S340.
3. Legrand M, Max A, Peigne V, et al. Survival in neutropenic patients with severe sepsis or septic shock. Crit Care Med 2012;20(1):43–9.
4. Dellinger RP, Levy MM, Rhodes A, et al. Surviving sepsis campaign: international guidelines for management of severe sepsis and septic shock: 2012. Crit Care Med 2013;41(2):580–637.
5. Flowers CR, Seidenfeld J, Bow EJ, et al. Antimicrobial prophylaxis and outpatient management of fever and neutropenia in adults treated for malignancy: American Society of Clinical Oncology clinical practice guideline. J Clin Oncol 2013;31(6): 794–810.
6. Keng MK, Sekeres MA. Febrile neutropenia in hematologic malignancies. Curr Hematol Malig Rep 2013;8:370–8.
7. Stewart AF. Hypercalcemia associated with cancer. N Engl J Med 2005;352: 373–9.

8. Grill V, Martin TJ. Hypercalcemia of malignancy. Rev Endocr Metab Disord 2000; 1:253–63.

9. Vassilopoulou-Sellin R, Newman BM, Taylor SH, et al. Incidence of hypercalcemia in patients with malignancy referred to a comprehensive cancer center. Cancer 1993;71:1309–12.

10. Sargent JT, Smith OP. Haematological emergencies managing hypercalcemia in adults and children with haematological disorders. Br J Haematol 2010;149: 465–77.

11. Wimalawansa SJ. Significance of plasma PTH-rp in patients with hypercalcemia of malignancy treated with bisphosphonate. Cancer 1994;73:2223–30.

12. Deftos LJ. Hypercalcemia in malignant and inflammatory diseases. Endocrinol Metab Clin North Am 2002;31:141–58.

13. Glass DA II, Patel MS, Karsenty G. A new insight into the formation of osteolytic lesions in multiple myeloma. N Engl J Med 2003;349:2479–80.

14. Brizendine K, Wells JM, Flanders SA, et al. Clinical problem solving. In search of.... N Engl J Med 2010;363:2249–54.

15. Behl D, Hendrickson AW, Moynihan TJ. Oncologic emergencies. Crit Care Clin 2010;26:181–205.

16. Gurney H, Grill V, Martin TJ. Parathyroid-related protein and response to pamidronate in tumour-induced hypercalcemia. Lancet 1993;341:1611–3.

17. Pi J, Kang Y, Smith M, et al. A review in the treatment of oncologic emergencies. J Oncol Pharm Pract 2015;1–14.

18. Lewis MA, Hendrickson AW, Moynihan TJ. Oncologic emergencies: pathophysiology, presentation, diagnosis, and treatment. CA Cancer J Clin 2011;61: 287–314.

19. Tanvetyanon T, Stiff PJ. Management of the adverse effects associated with intravenous bisphosphonates. Ann Oncol 2006;17:897–907.

20. Kacprowicz RF, Lloyd JD. Electrolyte complications of malignancy. Emerg Med Clin North Am 2009;27:257–69.

21. Gralow JR. Bisphosphonate risks and benefits: finding a balance. J Clin Oncol 2010;28:4873–6.

22. Wang CC, Chen YC, Shiang JC, et al. Hypercalcemic crisis successfully treated with prompt calcium-free hemodialysis. Am J Emerg Med 2009;27:1174.e1–3.

23. Pelosof LC, Gerber DE. Paraneoplastic syndromes: an approach to diagnosis and treatment. Mayo Clin Proc 2010;85:838–54.

24. Ljunghall S. Use of clodronate and calcitonin in hypercalcemia due to malignancy. Recent Results Cancer Res 1989;116:18–9.

25. Dumon JC, Magritte A, Body JJ. Nasal human calcitonin for tumor induced hypercalcemia. Calcif Tissue Int 1992;72:424–8.

26. Binstock ML, Mundy GR. Effect of calcitonin and glucocorticoids in combination on the hypercalcemia of malignancy. Ann Intern Med 1980;93:269–72.

27. Arseneau JC, Canellos GP, Banks PM, et al. American Burkitt's lymphoma: a clinicopathologic study of 30 cases. Clinical factors relating to prolonged survival. Am J Med 1975;58:314–21.

28. Annemans L, Moeremans K, Lamotte M, et al. Incidence, medical resource utilization and costs of hyperuricemia and tumour lysis syndrome in patients with acute leukemia and non-Hodgkin's lymphoma in four European countries. Leuk Lymphoma 2003;44:77–83.

29. McCroskey RD, Mosher DF, Spencer CD, et al. Acute tumor lysis syndrome in patients treated for refractory chronic lymphocytic leukemia with short-course,

high-dose cytosine arabinoside, cisplatin, and etoposide. Cancer 1990;66: 246–50.

30. Nomdedéu J, Martino R, Sureda A, et al. Acute tumor lysis syndrome complicating conditioning therapy for bone marrow transplantation in a patient with chronic lymphocytic leukemia. Bone Marrow Transplant 1994;13:659–60.

31. Bocca RV, Longo DL, Lieber ML, et al. Multiple recurrences of acute tumor lysis syndrome in an indolent non-Hodgkin's lymphoma. Cancer 1985;56:2295–7.

32. Gomez GA, Han T. Acute tumor lysis syndrome in prolymphocytic leukemia. Arch Intern Med 1987;147:375–6.

33. Cheson BD, Frame JN, Vena D, et al. Tumor lysis syndrome: an uncommon complication of fludarabine therapy of chronic lymphocytic leukemia. J Clin Oncol 1998;16:2313–20.

34. Howard S, Jones D, Pui C. The tumor lysis syndrome. N Engl J Med 2011;364: 1844–54.

35. Milka D, Ahmad S, Guruvayoorappan C. Tumor lysis syndrome: implications for cancer therapy. Asian Pac J Cancer Prev 2012;13:3555–60.

36. Cairo M, Bishop M. Tumor lysis syndrome: new therapeutic strategies and classification. Br J Haematol 2004;127:3–11.

37. Coiffer B, Altman A, Pui CH, et al. Guidelines for the management of pediatric and adult tumor lysis syndrome: an evidence-based review. J Clin Oncol 2008;26: 2767–78.

38. McBride A, Westervelt P. Recognizing and managing the expanded risk of tumor lysis syndrome in hematologic and solid malignancies. J Hematol Oncol 2012;5: 75–85.

39. Jones DP, Mahmoud H, Chesney RW. Tumor lysis syndrome: pathogenesis and management. Pediatr Nephrol 1995;9:206–12.

40. Andreoli SP, Clark JH, McGuire WA, et al. Purine excretion during tumor lysis in children with acute lymphocytic leukemia receiving allopurinol: relationship to acute renal failure. J Pediatr 1986;109:292–8.

41. Silverman P, Distelhorst CW. Metabolic emergencies in clinical oncology. Semin Oncol 1989;16:504–15.

42. Krakoff IH, Meyer RL. Prevention of hyperuricemia in leukemia and lymphoma. Use of allopurinol, a xanthine oxidase inhibitor. JAMA 1965;193:1–6.

43. Spector T. Inhibition of urate production by allopurinol. Biochem Pharmacol 1977; 26:355–8.

44. Holdsworth M, Nguyen P. Role of i.v. allopurinol and rasburicase in tumor lysis syndrome. Am J Health Syst Pharm 2003;60:2213–24.

45. Elitek [Package Insert]. Bridgewater (NJ): Sanofi-aventis; 2007.

46. McCurdy M, Shanholtz C. Oncologic emergencies. Crit Care Med 2012;40: 2212–22.

47. Ngugi NN, McLigeyo SP, Kayima JK. Treatment of hyperkalemia by altering the transcellular gradient in patients with renal failure: effect of various therapeutic approaches. East Afr Med J 1997;74:503–9.

48. Allon M, Dunlay R, Copkney C. Nebulized albuterol for acute hyperkalemia in patients on hemodialysis. Ann Intern Med 1989;110:426–9.

An Overview of Hematopoietic Stem Cell Transplantation

Carolyn M. Canonica, MMSc, PA-C*

KEYWORDS

- Bone marrow transplantation • Hematopoietic stem cell transplantation (HSCT)
- Peripheral blood stem cell transplantation (PBSCT) • Autologous transplant
- Allogeneic transplant • Complications of transplant

KEY POINTS

- Outline the stem cell transplantation process, from stem cell collection and pretransplant conditioning through post-transplant care, with a strong focus on post-transplant complications.
- Describe variables of stem cell transplant, including conditioning regimen, donor type, stem cell source, stem cell product manipulation, and immunosuppressant regimen.
- Introduce common medications used as prophylaxis and treatment in stem cell transplant patients during periods of neutropenia.
- Discuss new areas of research in the stem cell transplant field.

INTRODUCTION

Three years into my career as an internal medicine physician assistant (PA), I transitioned into the field of oncology, joining the Adult Bone Marrow Transplant Service at Memorial Sloan Kettering Cancer Center. Although I found my internal medicine background instrumental in the care of my bone marrow transplantation patients, my knowledge of stem cell transplantation was initially lacking. Like most PAs, I was not exposed to the bone marrow transplantation field during PA school due to the generalized nature of the medical education. The aim of this article is to expose primary care and oncology clinicians alike to this fascinating specialty by introducing core principles of bone marrow transplantation.

Note: hematopoietic stem cell transplantation (HSCT) is used in place of bone marrow transplantation in this article.

Disclosure Statement: The author has nothing to disclose.
Adult Bone Marrow Transplant Service, Department of Medicine, Memorial Sloan Kettering Cancer Center, 1275 York Avenue, New York, NY 10065, USA
* 104 Herman Boulevard, Franklin Square, New York, NY 11010.
E-mail addresses: canonicc@mskcc.org; carolyn.canonica@gmail.com

Physician Assist Clin 1 (2016) 409–418
http://dx.doi.org/10.1016/j.cpha.2016.03.006
physicianassistant.theclinics.com

INDICATION FOR TRANSPLANT

For patients whose hematologic malignancies and marrow disorders cannot be cured with conventional therapy, such as chemotherapy, radiation, or immunotherapy, HSCT provides a promising, potentially life-saving alternative treatment plan.[1] HSCT is a procedure by which diseased bone marrow is eradicated and replaced with healthy stem cells, which serve as progenitors for new, functional bone marrow and the re-establishment of normal hematopoiesis.[1]

Disease-free long-term survival is the ultimate goal of HSCT.[1] Outcomes are affected by myriad factors, including patient age and comorbidities, disease characteristics and prior therapy, conditioning regimen, stem cell source/donor variabilities, and graft-versus-host disease (GVHD) prophylaxis regimen.[1]

TYPES OF HEMATOPOIETIC STEM CELL TRANSPLANTATION

An autologous (auto) stem cell transplant requires patients to donate their own stem cells before undergoing high-dose chemotherapy.[1] These cells are taken either directly from the bone marrow via bone marrow harvest or, less invasively, via apheresis from the peripheral blood. Once obtained, these cells are frozen and later infused back into the patient, serving as a stem cell rescue after myeloablative conditioning regimens.[1] Autotransplants enable a patient's bone marrow to recover after high-dose chemotherapy. Although they confer a higher risk of relapse due to possible tumor contamination of rescue stem cells, autotransplants are associated with a lower risk of post-transplant complications.[1] They also eliminate the need for a donor search, HLA matching, or immune suppression. Autotransplants are commonly used for multiple myeloma, lymphomas, and testicular cancer.[1]

Allogeneic (allo) transplants require donation of stem cells from a donor, not from the patient. Related donors, in particular siblings, are preferable given the higher degree of histocompatibility between donor and patient.[1] Histocompatibility, which is determined by how closely a donor's HLA genes match those of the patient, is also used to determine a suitable unrelated donor for patients without a sibling match.[2] If a matched related donor (MRD) or matched unrelated donor (MUD) cannot be found, the patient becomes a candidate for transplantation using a mismatched unrelated donor or stem cells from an umbilical cord blood unit.[1,2] As the degree of histocompatibility between donor and patient increases, the risk of GVHD or graft failure decreases.[2]

The goal of an allotransplant is engraftment of donor cells that serves as the basis for the patient's new immune system. This new immune system, ideally free of disease, views the patient's residual tumor cells as foreign, initiating an immunologic attack known as the graft-versus-tumor (GVT) effect.[1] Allotransplants are commonly used in patients with leukemias, such as acute myeloid leukemia and chronic lymphoblastic leukemia.[1] Patients with myelodysplastic syndrome (MDS), follicular lymphoma, and aplastic anemia may also be candidates for allo-HSCT.[1]

STEM CELL COLLECTION

Sources of stem cells used for autotransplants and allotransplants include peripheral blood, bone marrow, and umbilical cord blood.[1] For this reason, the term, bone marrow transplantation, has been replaced by HSCT, because bone marrow is no longer used as the sole source of hematopoietic stem cells.[3] Today, peripheral blood stem cell collection via apheresis has supplanted bone marrow harvesting as the most common method by which to procure stem cells.[3] Peripheral blood stem cell transplantation, compared with bone marrow transplantation, not only is easier on the donor but also results in decreased time to engraftment for the patient.[4] Its major disadvantage, however, is its association with higher rates of chronic GVHD.[5] This increased GVHD risk is thought to be due to the larger concentration of CD3$^+$ T cells in peripheral blood stem cell products than in bone marrow products.[5]

Bone marrow is harvested from an autotransplant donor or allotransplant donor through needle aspirations from the posterior iliac crest, anterior iliac crest, or sternum.[1] Umbilical cord blood products are collected from the umbilical cord at the time of delivery.[1] Peripheral blood stem cells, on the other hand, can only be collected after administration of a hematopoietic growth factor, such as granulocyte colony-stimulating factor or plerixafor (Mozobil).[6] Granulocyte colony-stimulating factor and plerixafor are agents used to mobilize stem cells, promoting their transfer from the bone marrow into the peripheral blood, where they can then be collected via apheresis.[6]

Regardless of source, all stem cell products must be cryopreserved, or frozen, to maintain viability, unless they are scheduled to be used within 48 hours.[1] Dimethyl sulfoxide (DMSO) is an agent commonly used for cryopreservation. Modification or processing of the sample may precede cryopreservation; for example, red blood cells or plasma can be removed to reduce the volume of the sample.[1]

CONDITIONING REGIMEN

The purpose of a conditioning regimen is to destroy a patient's tumor cells prior to administration of the stem cell product.[1] Conditioning regimens range in intensity from myeloablative (high-dose regimens that completely destroy the bone marrow) to nonmyeloablative (lower-dose regimens that induce myelosuppression without destroying the bone marrow).[1] Nonmyeloablative regimens are more commonly used in patients with advanced age, comorbidities, history of prior HSCT, or malignancies that are either indolent or in remission.[1]

Ultimately, the goal of all conditioning regimens is to induce sufficient immunosuppression to prevent graft rejection while simultaneously balancing the risk of GVHD. Higher-dose chemotherapy regimens decrease a patient's risk of graft rejection and relapse, but they may increase morbidity and the risk of severe early GVHD.[1] One study found the incidence of toxic effects similar for standard and reduced-intensity conditioning[7]; however, the study participants were all younger than 60 years of age, with acute myeloid leukemia in first complete remission, so these results are not generalizable to the stem cell transplant population at large.[7]

The side effects and complications of conditioning regimens vary depending on the agents used. Carmustine, busulfan, cyclophosphamide, and melphalan are all alkylating agents.[1] Carmustine is known to cause pulmonary and renal toxicities. Seizure prophylaxis is recommended with busulfan given its neurotoxic effects. Cyclophosphamide can cause hemorrhagic cystitis, syndrome of inappropriate antidiuretic hormone secretion (SIADH), and cardiomyopathy.[1] Melphalan is known to cause significant mucositis, or ulceration and inflammation of the mucous membranes of the digestive tract.[8] Total body irradiation (TBI) is often used in conjunction with chemotherapy for conditioning, particularly for patients with certain leukemias or with central nervous system involvement. Patients receiving TBI often experience thyroid dysfunction, acute pneumonitis (diffuse alveolar hemorrhage), and gonadal failure (infertility).[1]

STEM CELL INFUSION

Once a patient has completed the conditioning regimen, stem cell infusion is the next step in the transplantation process. Before cryopreserved stem cells are infused into a patient, they are thawed quickly in a warm water bath.[9] Although many patients tolerate stem cell infusions well, side effects, such as fever, hypervolemia, and DMSO toxicity, can occur.[9] A fever should prompt collection of both blood cultures and stem cell product culture to rule out bacteremia and bacterial contamination of the product, respectively.[1] Hypervolemia can be treated with diuretics and by decreasing the rate of stem cell infusion.[1]

DMSO toxicity can result in an array of adverse reactions, including hemodynamic instability, nausea and vomiting, headache, cardiac arrhythmias, acute renal failure, and encephalopathy.[9] For this reason, stem cell products are sometimes washed via centrifugation prior to infusion in an attempt to limit the amount of DMSO a patient receives.[9] Concerns for stem cell loss, injury, and contamination in the DMSO removal process have prompted research into new washing methods.[9]

NEUTROPENIC PERIOD AND SUBSEQUENT IMMUNE RECOVERY (ENGRAFTMENT)

After stem cell infusion, patients are monitored closely as they await engraftment of their donor cells. Engraftment signifies replacement of the innate immune system by the donor graft.[1] A patient has achieved engraftment when the absolute neutrophil count is greater than 500 cells/μL on 2 consecutive days or 1000 cells/μL on 1 day.[1]

Time to engraftment varies depending on the type of transplant (autotransplant vs allotransplant) and the stem cell source (peripheral blood vs bone marrow vs umbilical cord).[1] Patients receiving peripheral blood HSCT engraft the soonest, followed by those receiving bone marrow HSCT, with cord blood recipients engrafting the slowest.[1] Autotransplants typically engraft more quickly than allotransplants; of 2 patients who have both received peripheral blood HSCT, the autotransplant engrafts at approximately days 9 to 12, whereas the allotransplant engrafts at approximately day 10 to 14.[1] GVHD prophylaxis can also have an impact on time to engraftment; methotrexate, for example, can lead to slower engraftment.[1]

Because patients are neutropenic while awaiting engraftment, infection prophylaxis is of utmost importance.[1] An expected consequence of transplant that is indicative of a suppressed or ablated immune system, neutropenia is defined as an absolute neutrophil count less than 1500 cells/μL.[10] The risk of clinically significant infection rises when the neutropenic period is of prolonged duration (>7 days) and/or classified as "severe" (absolute neutrophil count <500 cells/μL).[10,11] Thus, anti-infective prophylaxis, in the form of antibiotic, antifungal, and antiviral medications, has become routine for HSCT patients.[10]

Blood cultures must be drawn if a patient develops a fever during the neutropenic period, and prophylactic anti-infectives are escalated to empiric broader-spectrum agents.[1] First-line therapy for febrile neutropenia includes a third-generation or fourth-generation cephalosporin; vancomycin may be added if a patient is colonized with methicillin-resistant *Staphylococcus aureus*, blood cultures are positive for gram-positive bacteria, and/or an indwelling catheter is suspected as the source of fever.[1]

Neutropenic fever is a major adverse event in cancer patients, and it remains a significant cause of morbidity and mortality in patients receiving HSCT.[12] Blood culture–confirmed bacteremia accounts for 10% to 30% of neutropenic fever cases.[12] Given the steady rise of multidrug-resistant organisms, like *Escherichia coli* and *Klebsiella pneumoniae*, this is particularly worrisome in the severely immune-compromised HSCT population, rendering culture-driven antibiotic therapy imperative.[12]

POSTENGRAFTMENT

Once engraftment has occurred and patients are deemed clinically stable for hospital discharge, preventative care at home becomes paramount to recovery.[1] In addition to routine hand washing and avoiding sick contacts, post-HSCT patients are advised to avoid travel, minimize contact with pets (specifically feces and litter boxes), and follow a low-microbial diet until adequate immune recovery.[1] Exposure to tobacco, soil, well water, construction sites, and crowded public areas is also strongly discouraged. To prevent bleeding, sexual activity must be avoided until the platelet count reaches 50,000, and condom use is essential to reduce risk of sexually transmitted pathogens.[1]

Vaccinations play a vital role in the long-term health of post-HSCT patients.[1] Although patients may have received vaccinations before transplant, antibody titers decline after transplant and may no longer offer optimal protection against disease. Vaccines are administered once a patient's immune system has fully recovered, which is usually between 1 to 2 years post-HSCT.[1] Inactivated vaccines, such as diphtheria and tetanus toxoids and pertussis vaccine; Haemophilus b conjugate vaccine; and inactivated poliovirus vaccine are initiated at 12 months post-HSCT.[1] Patients require lifelong, annual influenza vaccination, and all household members should also be vaccinated prior to the start of peak influenza season.[1]

In contrast, live-attenuated vaccines such as the measles, mumps, and rubella virus vaccine (MMR), cannot be given until at least 2 years after transplant.[1] The live-attenuated varicella-zoster virus (VZV), or shingles, vaccine is contraindicated in post-transplant patients. Because shingles is common after HSCT, with an incidence up to 50% to 60%, it is imperative that patients' family members and household contacts are vaccinated against VZV.[1] Live vaccines are always contraindicated in patients with chronic GVHD who require systemic immunosuppressant medications.[1]

COMPLICATIONS OF TRANSPLANT

Not all HSCT patients follow a similar trajectory after engraftment. Post-transplant complications manifest differently, and vary in severity, based on individualized factors.[1] A patient's age and preexisting comorbidities, transplant type, stem cell source, degree of donor/recipient HLA match (for allotransplants), prophylactic anti-infective and immunosuppressant medications, conditioning regimen, and number of days post-transplant are just a few variables to consider when diagnosing and treating complications.[1]

Infection

Despite efforts to prevent infection with prophylactic agents, HSCT patients remain at high risk for infection, even months to years post-transplant.[1] Infections, in particular those of fungal and viral origin, cause significant morbidity and mortality for HSCT patients, independent of graft source.[13]

From day 0 (day of stem cell infusion) to day 30 (30 days after stem cell infusion), patients are particularly vulnerable to infections related to neutropenia and the conditioning regimen. These infections can manifest as gastrointestinal or catheter-associated bacteremias or as invasive fungal infections, such as aspergillosis.[1] Antibiotic prophylaxis with fluoroquinolones has been shown to reduce mortality in afebrile neutropenic patients.[10] For antifungal prophylaxis, patients may receive fluconazole, which covers *Candida*, or voriconazole, a broader-spectrum antifungal agent with activity against *Aspergillus*.[10]

Beyond day 30, patients become more susceptible to various viral pathogens and opportunistic infections.[1] Cytomegalovirus, Epstein-Barr virus, adenovirus, and herpes viruses are common nonrespiratory viruses that afflict post-transplant patients.[1] Pancytopenia often results from these viral infections, which only amplifies a patient's risk of additional infections.[14] Acyclovir is often used as antiviral prophylaxis and continued for several months after discontinuation of immunosuppression.[1] One study recommends the continuation of acyclovir prophylaxis for up to a year post-autotransplant to prevent herpes simplex virus and VZV.[15]

Pneumocystis jiroveci pneumonia (PCP) and toxoplasmosis are 2 opportunistic infections that are commonly seen after HSCT.[1] Medication to prevent PCP should be initiated after engraftment, within 30 days after transplant.[13] Trimethoprim/sulfamethoxazole (Bactrim) is the drug of choice for PCP and also provides protection against *T. gondii*.[1]

Patients who are asymptomatically colonized with toxigenic *Clostridium difficile* prior to HSCT are at risk of developing *C. difficile* infection, a leading cause of infectious diarrhea and a major cause of morbidity in HSCT recipients.[16] The potential for nosocomial transmission of *C. difficile* to previously noncolonized HSCT patients makes infection control particularly challenging.[16] In addition to diarrhea, at least one-third to one-half of patients with *C. difficile* infection also develop fever and abdominal pain.[16] Metronidazole (Flagyl) and vancomycin are 2 agents used to treat *C. difficile* infection.[16]

Engraftment Syndrome

Engraftment syndrome (ES) should be strongly considered in patients who develop the triad of generalized rash, peripheral and/or pulmonary (noncardiogenic) edema, and high fevers in the first 2 weeks after HSCT or at the time of engraftment.[1] Transient encephalopathy, along with hepatic and renal dysfunction, can also be seen with ES.[17] Although the etiology of ES is poorly understood, proinflammatory cytokine production that accompanies neutrophil recovery is thought to play a role, considering the resolution of symptoms once immune reconstitution has been achieved.[17] ES is a diagnosis of exclusion made only after GVHD, infection, drug reaction, and transfusion-related acute lung injury have been ruled out. ES is diagnosed clinically and treated with corticosteroids.[1] The validity of ES as a diagnosis remains controversial, because some experts believe that ES is actually an early manifestation of acute GVHD.[17]

Graft-Versus-Host Disease

One of the leading causes of morbidity and mortality among allo-HSCT recipients, GVHD occurs in the presence of histocompatibility mismatch between donor and host.[1] GVHD is an immunologically mediated process during which the graft (donor) T cells attack host antigens that they view as foreign, resulting in significant tissue injury.[18] The gastrointestinal tract, skin, and liver are the 3 organ systems most commonly affected by GVHD, although new research points to reproductive and neurologic complications as well.[18] Although GVHD is one of the most feared complications of transplant, it has been associated with beneficial GVT effects.[1]

GVHD prophylaxis takes the form of either immunosuppressant medication or graft manipulation (T-cell depletion).[1] Agents such as methotrexate, sirolimus, mycophenolate mofetil, and calcineurin inhibitors (tacrolimus or cyclosporin) are used in various combinations as GVHD prophylactic regimens.[1] Graft manipulation, in the form of T-cell depletion of the donor stem cell product prior to transplantation, can be used independently of or in conjunction with immunosuppressive regimens to prevent

GVHD.[1] Although T-cell depletion transplants are associated with decreased transplant-related mortality due to lower risks of GVHD, they are also associated with an increased rate of disease relapse post-transplant.[1]

The diagnosis of chronic GVHD can be made using 1 of 2 pathways: (1) the presence of 1 diagnostic manifestation (pathognomonic sign on physical examination); or (2) the presence of at least 1 distinctive manifestation (supportive, but not pathognomonic, sign on physical examination) in addition to a diagnosis-confirming laboratory result, radiology finding, or biopsy in the same or another organ.[1] Systemic steroids are the first-line treatment of chronic GVHD.[1]

Sinusoidal Obstruction Syndrome

Sinusoidal obstruction syndrome (SOS), formerly known as venoocclusive disease, is a well-established, potentially lethal complication of the high-dose chemotherapy conditioning regimens given prior to HSCT.[19] In SOS, small hepatic vessels become obstructed due to a complex pathophysiologic process characterized by endothelial injury and hepatocellular necrosis.[1] As the venules of the liver fibrose, patients with SOS can develop severe hepatic congestion and eventual organ compromise or failure.[1] SOS occurs in up to 12% of autotransplant patients and 40% of allotransplant patients.[20]

High-dose chemotherapy, TBI, preexisting liver disease, and history of prior HSCT are all important risk factors for SOS.[1] The syndrome has also been associated with prior iron overload, recurrent fevers, and high-dose intravenous immunoglobulin.[1] Given the large number of risk factors in HSCT patients, ursodiol is used as SOS prophylaxis.[1]

The classic triad of jaundice, ascites or weight gain of unclear etiology, and painful hepatomegaly can be used to clinically diagnose SOS.[21] Hyperbilirubinemia, along with a Doppler ultrasound revealing portal vein dilation, ascites, and gallbladder wall thickening in the absence of cholangitis, supports the diagnosis.[1] Liver biopsy remains the gold standard for diagnosing SOS.[1]

Treatment of mild to moderate SOS is largely supportive by way of fluid restriction and diuretic therapy.[20] Conversely, severe SOS, which results in multisystem organ failure and progressive hepatorenal syndrome, portends a grave prognosis and requires aggressive treatment.[20] One large study demonstrated approximately 15% to 30% survival on day 100 for 4300 patients with severe SOS.[21] Defibrotide, a DNA adenosine receptor agonist that induces vasodilation and repairs sinusoidal endothelial cells, is currently the most promising drug used as treatment of severe SOS.[20]

Graft Rejection and Graft Failure

Graft rejection and graft failure are serious complications of HSCT. When a recipient's residual immune system views donor stem cells as foreign, it launches an immunologic response known as graft rejection.[1] Rejection is characterized by the presence of recipient T cells and the absence of donor cells in the blood and bone marrow.[22] Graft rejection manifests as either lack of initial engraftment of donor cells or loss of the donor graft after an initial successful engraftment.[22]

Graft failure, on the other hand, is not immune mediated, although graft rejection can precipitate eventual graft failure.[22] Graft failure results from inadequate stem cell dose or viability.[1] An important distinction between graft failure and graft rejection can be made using chimerism testing, or engraftment analysis that uses polymerase chain reaction techniques to determine the genetic makeup of a patient's hematopoietic cells[22]; a patient experiencing graft failure has 100% donor T cells (and no recipient T cells) on blood or marrow chimerism studies but has not achieved hematologic recovery.[1]

The prevalence of graft rejection increases as the degree of donor/recipient HLA mismatch increases and, therefore, occurs more frequently in patients receiving unrelated or mismatched transplants.[1] Reduced-intensity chemotherapy conditioning regimens, as opposed to myeloablative regimens, are also associated with a greater risk of graft rejection due to the possibility that the abnormal immune system is not completely eradicated prior to HSCT.[1] Graft failure, on the other hand, is induced by drug toxicity, septicemia, and/or viral infections, such as human herpesvirus 6, cytomegalovirus, and VZV.[22]

Graft rejection is treated with the administration of a second stem cell product with a lesser degree of HLA mismatch, preferably after a highly immunosuppressive conditioning regimen.[1] Graft failure that is "full donor" by chimerism analysis is also treated with the infusion of a second stem cell product, ideally a T-cell–depleted product to reduce the risk of GVHD.[1] Even when treated properly, graft failure is associated with a high mortality rate due to the risk of infections during the prolonged neutropenic period.[1]

AREAS OF RESEARCH

Long-term disease-free survival is the primary goal of HSCT.[1] Determined by variables such as patient age, diagnosis, disease stage, and transplant factors, 5-year disease-free survival can range from 5% to 80% for HSCT patients,[1] necessitating improved methods to bolster overall outcomes. Although allotransplants may have curative potential, some patients are not eligible for these transplants given the lack of a suitable matched donor.[23] The availability of MUDs for members of underrepresented minorities, such as African Americans, is particularly low.[24]

In light of this issue, HLA-haploidentical transplants are gaining ground and have produced promising results, specifically in patients with leukemia and lymphoma.[23] The donor for an HLA-haploidentical (partially HLA-mismatched) transplant is a first-degree relative who matches the patient at only 1 HLA haplotype.[1,23] A patient's biological children, parents, and siblings are all potential HLA-haploidentical donors, and siblings have a 50% chance of being a suitable donor.[24] One transplant center identified a haploidentical donor for greater than 95% of their patients, whereas only 50% to 60% of patients on average are found to have a suitable MRD or MUD.[24]

Although they may provide rapid acquisition of a greater number of potential donors, haploidentical transplants have significant drawbacks.[24] Due to bidirectional alloreactivity (ie, the interplay of direct recognition of allo-HLA by HLA-specific alloantibodies and T cells and indirect T-cell recognition), haploidentical transplants have been associated with delayed engraftment, graft failure, transplant-related mortality, and severe GVHD.[24] For the same reason, however, haploidentical transplants have also been shown to produce a more potent GVT effect than is induced by an HLA-matched graft.[24]

Currently, allotransplant HSCT using a MRD produces the best outcomes.[24] The difference in 5-year disease-free survival rates, however, among allotransplants using MRDs, MUDs, umbilical cord blood, and HLA-haploidentical donors is narrowing.[24] Given the incidence of relapse with haploidentical HSCT, research is ongoing to improve cellular therapies (using natural killer cells or donor chimeric antigen receptor T cells) and maintenance chemotherapy regimens.[23]

HOW TO BECOME A STEM CELL DONOR

Finding a suitable donor is the first step toward a successful allo–stem cell transplant. Because 70% of eligible transplant patients do not have an MRD, they must rely solely on donations from volunteers.[25] Donors with diverse ethnic and racial heritages are especially needed, because the likelihood of donor-patient HLA match increases with the degree of ethnic and racial similarity.[25]

The National Marrow Donor Program (NMDP) is an excellent resource for potential donors (ages 18–44) who are interested in joining the bone marrow registry, learning about the donation and transplantation process, or organizing donor registry drives in their communities.[25] The NMDP provides medical teams from transplant centers worldwide with access to approximately 25 million potential donors and 600,000 cord blood units.[25] The current likelihood of finding a MUD through the NMDP ranges from 66% to 97%, depending on ethnic and racial background.[25] This number can only increase if more volunteers join the registry.

SUMMARY

HSCT is an ever-growing field that has improved outcomes for patients whose blood and marrow disorders are refractory to conventional therapies. In addition to the well-established procedures for auto-HSCT and conventional allo-HSCT, transplants using umbilical cord blood and haploidentical stem cell products now serve as promising options for patients who would otherwise be ineligible for HSCT. Post-transplant complications, such as infections and GVHD, continue to be the cause of significant morbidity and mortality, although hopefully these will improve in conjunction with continued advances in the field.

REFERENCES

1. Antin JH, Raley DY. Manual of stem cell and bone marrow transplantation. 1st edition. New York: Cambridge University Press; 2009.
2. Soiffer RJ. Hematopoietic stem cell transplantation. 2nd edition. Totowa (NJ): Humana; 2008. p. 19, 24, 25.
3. Lopez-Larrea C. Stem cell transplantation. New York: Springer Science and Business Media; 2012. p. 121, 126, 128, 129.
4. The promise of stem cells. NIH stem cell information home page. Bethesda (MD): National Institutes of Health, U.S. Department of Health and Human Services; 2015. Available at. http://stemcells.nih.gov/info/basics. Accessed November 30, 2015.
5. Cutler C, Antin JH. Peripheral blood stem cells for allogeneic transplantation: a review. Stem Cells 2001;19(2):108–17.
6. Cashen A, Lopez S, Gao F, et al. A phase II study of plerixafor (AMD3100) plus G-CSF for autologous hematopoietic progenitor cell mobilization in patients with Hodgkin Lymphoma. Biol Blood Marrow Transplant 2008;14(11):1253–61.
7. Bornhauser M, Kienast J, Trenschel R, et al. Reduced-intensity conditioning versus standard conditioning before allogeneic haemopoietic cell transplantation in patients with acute myeloid leukaemia in first complete remission: a prospective, open-label randomised phase 3 trial. Lancet Oncol 2012;13(10): 1035–44.
8. Grazziutti ML, Dong L, Miceli MH, et al. Oral mucositis in myeloma patients undergoing melphalan-based autologous stem cell transplantation: incidence, risk factors and a severity predictive model. Bone Marrow Transplant 2006;38(7): 501–6.
9. Shu Z, Heimfeld S, Gao D. Hematopoietic stem cell transplantation with cryopreserved grafts: adverse reactions after transplantation and cryoprotectant removal prior to infusion. Bone Marrow Transplant 2014;49(4):469–76.

10. Villafuerte-Gutierrez P, Villalon L, Losa JE, et al. Treatment of febrile neutropenia and prophylaxis in hematologic malignancies: a critical review and update. Adv Hematol 2014;2014:986938.

11. Tomblyn M, Chiller T, Einsele H, et al. Guidelines for preventing infectious complications among hematopoietic cell transplant recipients: a global perspective. Bone Marrow Transplant 2009;15(10):453–5.

12. Wang L, Wang Y, Fan X, et al. Prevalence of resistant gram-negative bacilli in bloodstream infection in febrile neutropenia patients undergoing hematopoietic stem cell transplantation: a Single Center Retrospective Cohort Study. Medicine (Baltimore) 2015;94(45):e1931.

13. Young JAH, Logan BR, Wu J, et al. Infections after transplantation of bone marrow or peripheral blood stem cells from unrelated donors. Biol Blood Marrow Transplant 2016;22(2):359–70. Clinical Trials Network Trial 0201.

14. Bilgrami S, Almeida GD, Quinn JJ, et al. Pancytopenia in allogeneic marrow transplant recipients: role of cytomegalovirus. Br J Haematol 1994;87(2):357–62.

15. Kawamura K, Hayakawa J, Akahoshi Y, et al. Low-dose acyclovir prophylaxis for the prevention of herpes simplex virus and varicella zoster virus diseases after autologous hematopoietic stem cell transplantation. Int J Hematol 2015;102(2): 230–7.

16. Jain T, Croswell C, Urday-Cornejo V, et al. Clostridium difficile colonization in hematopoietic stem cell transplant recipients: a prospective study of the epidemiology and outcomes involving toxigenic and nontoxigenic strains. Biol Blood Marrow Transplant 2015;15:497–8.

17. Cornell RF, Hari P, Drobyski WR. Engraftment syndrome after autologous stem cell transplantation: an update unifying the definition and management approach. Biol Blood Marrow Transplant 2015;21(12):2061–8.

18. Teshima T, Reddy P, Zeiser R. Acute graft-versus-host disease: novel biological insights. Biol Blood Marrow Transplant 2016;22(1):11–6.

19. Rubbia-Brandt L. Sinusoidal obstruction syndrome. Clin Liver Dis 2010;14(4): 651–68.

20. Triplett BM, Kuttab HI, Kang G, et al. Escalation to high-dose defibrotide in patients with hepatic veno-occlusive disease. Biol Blood Marrow Transplant 2015; 21(12):2148–53.

21. Yakushijin K, Atsuta Y, Doki N, et al. Sinusoidal obstruction syndrome after allogeneic hematopoietic stem cell transplantation: incidence, risk factors, and outcomes. Bone Marrow Transplant 2015;51(3):403–9.

22. Mattsson J, Ringdén O, Storb R. Graft failure after allogeneic hematopoietic cell transplantation. Biol Blood Marrow Transplant 2008;14(1):165–70.

23. Showel M, Fuchs EJ. Recent developments in HLA-haploidentical transplantations. Best Pract Res Clin Haematol 2015;28(2–3):141–6.

24. Fuchs EJ. Haploidentical transplantation for hematologic malignancies: where do we stand? Hematology Am Soc Hematol Educ Program 2012;2012(1):230–6.

25. National Marrow Donor Program website. Published 1996-2015. Available at: https://bethematch.org. Accessed January 27, 2016.

Management of Graft-Versus-Host Disease

Jerrad M. Stoddard, MA, MS, PA-C*, Tamera Plair, MS, PA-C,
Yvonne H. Jee, MS, PA-C

KEYWORDS

- Allogeneic stem cell transplant • Graft-versus-host disease • Acute • Chronic
- Management • Complications

KEY POINTS

- Graft-versus-host disease (GVHD) is a major cause of late nonrelapse mortality in allogeneic hematopoietic stem cell transplant recipients.
- GVHD is a complex, polymorphic disease that affects numerous organ systems and warrants prompt evaluation, management, and referral.
- GVHD treatment requires close monitoring for disease response, drug trough levels, and side effects.
- There are numerous complications that can occur from GVHD and its management, such as drug toxicity/side effects, renal insufficiency, endocrinopathies, and secondary malignancies.
- Primary care providers should be familiar with screening allogeneic stem cell transplant recipients for GVHD, monitoring drug levels and side effects, and screening for complications.

INTRODUCTION

Hematopoietic stem cell transplant (HSCT) possesses the potential to cure many malignant and nonmalignant hematologic diseases. Autologous HSCT uses cells collected from the patient to treat many lymphomas, multiple myeloma, and germ cell tumors. Allogeneic HSCT (allo-HSCT) includes all transplants in which the patient receives donor stem cells after a chemotherapeutic conditioning regimen. Donor stem cells are collected from family members (eg, siblings, parents, children), voluntary unrelated donors, and umbilical cord blood units. Between 2006 and 2014, there were 400,301 allo-HSCTs performed worldwide.[1] The curative potential of allo-HSCT was first reported in the 1950s when leukemic mice were irradiated before receiving allogeneic bone marrow transplants and were noted to have successful disease eradication; however, leukemic mice receiving stem cells from identical twins had persistent

Disclosures: None.
Department of Stem Cell Transplantation and Cellular Therapy, The University of Texas MD Anderson Cancer Center, 1515 Holcombe Boulevard, Unit 423, Houston, TX 77030, USA
* Corresponding author.
E-mail address: jstoddard@mdanderson.org

Physician Assist Clin 1 (2016) 419–433
http://dx.doi.org/10.1016/j.cpha.2016.03.007
2405-7991/16/$ – see front matter © 2016 Elsevier Inc. All rights reserved.

disease, suggesting a graft-versus-tumor effect caused by the genetic differences of donor cells.[2] Subsequently, the development of novel strategies that use nonmyeloablative conditioning regimens, donor leukocyte infusions, umbilical cord blood transplantations, and haplo-identical transplantation has helped expand the immunotherapeutic benefits of allo-HSCT.[3] Despite these advances, allo-HSCT is often associated with a major intrinsic complication: graft-versus-host disease (GVHD).

GVHD occurs when the graft (donor cells) recognizes the host (recipient) as foreign and launches an immune attack against the host cells causing organ dysfunction and/or failure. There are three defining factors that must be present for GVHD to develop: (1) the donor graft must contain immune competent cells; (2) the host must express tissue antigens not present in the donor (also described as histocompatibility differences); and (3) the host must be unable to reject or eliminate transplanted donor cells.[4] Although the pathophysiology of GVHD remains to be fully elucidated, GVHD occurs in three phases.[5] First, the conditioning regimen for the allo-HSCT damages host tissues, which causes the release of proinflammatory cytokines. Then upon engraftment of donor cells and immune reconstitution, donor T lymphocytes are stimulated by circulating cytokines and interact with various antigens on host cells, which leads to T-cell activation and initiation of immune response.[6] One of the most important proteins recognized by donor T cells are human leukocyte antigens (HLAs) encoded by the major histocompatibility complex. Class I HLA (A, B, C) proteins are expressed on all nucleated cells of the body in various densities. Class II proteins (DR, DQ, and DP) are mainly expressed on hematopoietic cells, but their expression is induced on many other cell types after inflammation or injury. After activation, donor-derived T cells proliferate and differentiate into effector cells, and activated T cells migrate to target tissues (ie, skin, liver, and gut) where they cause destruction through direct cytotoxic activity and recruitment of other leukocytes.

Risk factors for development of GVHD have been extensively studied. The degree of HLA mismatching is the most important risk factor because the donor immune system is more likely to recognize recipient cells with more antigen mismatch.[7] Furthermore, the source of donor stem cells is a critical factor.[7–9] Peripheral blood stem cells contain donor T lymphocytes, which directly mediate the development of GVHD. However, stem cells derived from umbilical cord blood units contain naive immune cells, which minimizes the risk of developing GVHD. Gender disparity also increases the risk of GVHD if a female donor is used for a male recipient.[7] This may be explained by minor histocompatibility antigens that are encoded by the Y chromosome in males, which would presumably increase reactivity of donor cells. These factors, among others, are carefully taken into account when selecting an optimal donor to mitigate the risk of GVHD.

GVHD can be divided into two general categories: acute (aGVHD) and chronic (cGVHD). Historically, GVHD occurring within the first 100 days after allo-HSCT was defined as aGVHD, and occurrence after Day 100 was classified as cGVHD.[10–12] However, the terminology was redefined by the National Institutes of Health Consensus group, which recognized that signs of aGVHD and cGVHD can occur irrespective of the arbitrary 100-day mark. According to the established criteria, aGVHD and cGVHD are distinguished by clinical manifestations and not by time after allo-HSCT.[13] These criteria were later updated in 2014 by the National Institutes of Health Consensus group.[14]

CLINICAL FEATURES OF ACUTE GRAFT-VERSUS-HOST DISEASE

aGVHD is a potentially life-threatening complication of allo-HSCT that requires prompt diagnosis and therapeutic intervention. Clinical manifestations, staging, and grading of aGVHD are based on the primary target organs affected: skin, liver, and gut.[10] Biopsies of the involved organ are important to confirm the diagnosis of aGVHD because the differential diagnoses are vast following allo-HSCT and include side effects from chemotherapy or medications, drug allergies, infection, and peptic ulcers.

The most common presentation of aGVHD of the skin is a pruritic, erythematous, maculopapular rash (**Fig. 1**). This can spread and become more confluent in nature and even progress to blistering and ulceration, often mimicking Stevens-Johnson syndrome.

aGVHD can also affect the upper and/or lower gastrointestinal (GI) tract. Anorexia, nausea, and vomiting may indicate upper GI involvement. Secretory voluminous diarrhea is the most common presentation of lower GI GVHD. Because the amount of diarrhea is the easiest and most objective quantitative measurement, this is used to assess severity and grade of GI GVHD.

Hepatic involvement of aGVHD rarely presents without either skin or gut manifestations. It usually presents as cholestasis with elevations in serum direct bilirubin and alkaline phosphatase. However, isolated elevation of transaminases can occur. The histopathology is not specific but often reveals portal infiltration with T lymphocytes and epithelial bile duct damage and/or degenerative changes.

aGVHD is staged by the degree of involvement of each organ followed by an overall grading score (**Table 1**). Overall grading of aGVHD is mild (I), moderate (II), severe (III), and very severe (IV). Severe (grade III) and very severe (grade IV) GVHD have a poor prognosis with a 5-year survival rate of 25% and 5%, respectively.[15]

CLINICAL FEATURES OF CHRONIC GRAFT-VERSUS-HOST DISEASE

cGVHD is a major cause of late nonrelapse mortality.[16] The disease is pleomorphic and affects numerous organs, including the skin (most commonly), GI tract, liver, lungs, oral cavity, eyes, and vaginal canal (**Fig. 2, Table 2**). cGVHD more frequently presents as a progression from aGVHD or with concurrent symptoms of aGVHD called overlap syndrome; however, it can arise with de novo onset. cGVHD often impacts quality of life. For example, patients with skin cGVHD may present with fascial involvement and have restricted range of motion or contractures, which can cause inabilities to perform simple tasks, such as opening a jar or brushing one's hair. cGVHD can also be precipitated by infections. For example, pulmonary cGVHD, also known as

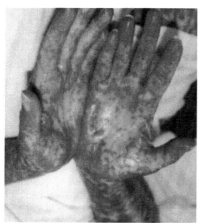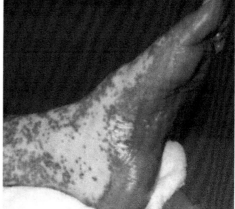

Fig. 1. Acute skin GVHD. Presents as a pruritic, maculopapular rash.

Table 1
Staging acute GVHD by organ system

Stage	Skin (% Body Surface Area)	Liver (Bilirubin mg/dL)	Gut (mL Stool Volume/d)
0	0	<2.0	<500
1	<25	2.0–2.9	>500
2	25–50	3.0–5.9	>1000
3	>50, generalized erythroderma	6.0–14.9	>1500
4	Bullae/desquamation	>15.0	>2000

Overall Grade of Acute GVHD by Glucksber	
Grade I	Stage 1 or 2 skin involvement; no liver or gut involvement
Grade II	Stage 1–3 skin involvement, stage 1 liver or gut involvement
Grade III	Stage 2 or 3 skin, liver, or gut involvement
Grade IV	Stage 1–4 skin involvement; stage 2–4 liver or gut involvement

bronchiolitis obliterans, is often incited by respiratory infections, most commonly parainfluenza and respiratory syncytial virus.[17] Assessing patients for cGVHD is challenging because the differential diagnosis is broad and patients may have subtle clinical presentation. For example, patients with pulmonary cGVHD may present

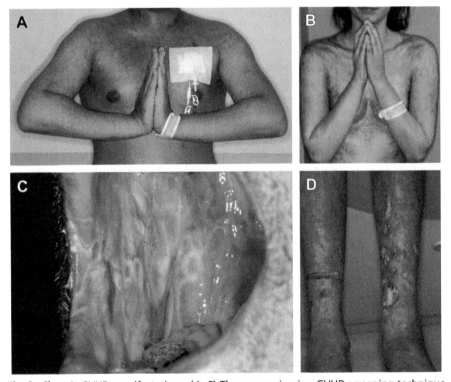

Fig. 2. Chronic GVHD manifestations. (*A, B*) The prayer sign is a GVHD screening technique to identify underlying fasciitis in patients. (*A*) Negative prayer sign. (*B*) Positive prayer sign with limited wrist dorsiflexion and proximal/distal interphalangeal extension. (*C*) Lichenoid changes of the buccal mucosa seen in oral cGVHD. (*D*) Bullous lesions of the lower extremities consistent with cGVHD of the skin.

Table 2
Overview of chronic GVHD manifestations

Organ System Involved	Symptoms	Physical Examination and Clinical Findings	Comments
Integumentary	Skin tightening, decreased range of motion, alopecia, nail dystrophy	Lichen planus, sclerosis, blisters, ulcerations, hypopigmentation/hyperpigmentation, restricted motion, contractures, longitudinal striations of nails, onycholysis/nail loss	Skin punch biopsy is recommended; histopathology demonstrates perivascular lymphocytic infiltration and apoptotic keratinocytes
Oral cavity	Xerostomia, oral sensitivity to spicy/acidic foods or toothpaste, dry/cracked lips	Lichen planus of the buccal mucosa, palatal mucoceles, ulcerations	—
Gastrointestinal	Dysphagia, anorexia, chronic nausea, malabsorptive symptoms	Weight loss, esophagogastroduodenoscopy may reveal esophageal strictures or webbing	—
Liver	Usually asymptomatic; may present with jaundice in advanced disease	Typically presents as cholestasis (elevated direct bilirubin and alkaline phosphatase); may present with transaminitis	Broad differential diagnosis including medication, infection, iron overload, GVHD; transjugular liver biopsy is recommended; histopathology demonstrates damage/loss of bile duct epithelial cells and piecemeal necrosis
Pulmonary	Dry cough, dyspnea, decreased exercise tolerance	Pulmonary function tests show obstructive pattern (FEV_1/FVC ratio <0.7; FEV_1 <75% predicted value; RV >120%); CT imaging shows air trapping or bronchiectasis	—
Eyes	Dry eyes, ocular irritation, foreign body sensation	Scleral injection, corneal ulceration, positive Schirmer test	Provider may quantify severity or response to treatment by number of eye drops used in a day
Genitalia	Dyspareunia, itching, burning, vaginal dryness/atrophy	Lichen planus of vaginal mucosa or penis, vaginal scarring or introital	—

Abbreviations: CT, computed tomography; FEV_1, forced expiratory volume in 1 second; FVC, forced vital capacity; RV, residual volume.

with decreased exercise tolerance or shortness of breath, suggesting a cardiac cause. Pulmonary function testing is the key screening/diagnostic tool and reveals an airflow obstruction pattern. Additionally, patients with liver cGVHD may present with acute elevation in liver enzymes, and the differential diagnosis includes drug-induced hepatotoxicity, infectious etiologies, biliary disease, and autoimmune disease.

The clinical presentation cGVHD is variable depending on the organ systems involved, and cGVHD can mimic autoimmune conditions, such as scleroderma and Sjögren syndrome. Thus, it is easily misdiagnosed. Therefore, it is imperative that general practitioners in the community are aware of cGVHD manifestations in allo-HSCT recipients and are capable of screening patients appropriately.

MANAGEMENT OF GRAFT-VERSUS-HOST DISEASE

Because GVHD is a multifaceted complication of allo-HSCT, prevention is critical and is a steep task in the transplant community. Immunosuppressive regimens are widely used for GVHD prevention and treatment. Calcineurin inhibitors, such as tacrolimus (Prograf), suppress the immune system by reducing the gene expression of many early cytokines including interleukin-2, tumor necrosis factor-α, and interferon-γ. Additionally, mammalian target of rapamycin inhibitors, such as sirolimus (Rapamune), inhibit the growth of hematopoietic and lymphoid cells. Both tacrolimus and sirolimus have a narrow therapeutic index (target range of 6–10 ng/mL). Once dosing is established early in the posttransplant setting, trough levels are monitored periodically to ensure that levels do not become supratherapeutic (ie, >10 ng/mL). There are a variety of methods used for GVHD prophylaxis in patients with allo-HSCT that vary from one transplant center to another. At our institution, we use tacrolimus, minidose methotrexate (Trexall), and posttransplant cyclophosphamide (Cytoxan) as preventative measures. We also aim to educate patients on prevention and potential triggering factors, such as sun exposure and infections. We maintain patients on GVHD prophylaxis for approximately 3–6 months posttransplant before considering initiating a taper. Despite these measures, a sizable number of patients develop GVHD. Even more challenging is the management of this entity because there is a spectrum of treatment options that are not standardized.

Management of Acute Graft-Versus-Host Disease

Grade II to IV aGVHD occurs in approximately 35% to 50% of patients who receive an allo-HSCT despite prophylaxis with immunosuppressive agents.[18] Treatment of GVHD ranges from topical treatments to comprehensive systemic therapies based on the degree of involvement (see **Table 1**). Limited or mild aGVHD includes single organ involvement or stage I/grade I classification. The management of grade I disease should include topical therapy and optimizing levels of calcineurin inhibitors without the need for additional systemic immunosuppression.[19]

In cutaneous aGVHD involving less than 50% body surface area (ie, grade I), topical management is initiated first, and there is a host of low- to high-potency topical corticosteroids (**Table 3**). Hydrocortisone and desonide cream are often used for the more sensitive regions, such as the face, axilla, and groin. The more potent steroids, such as triamcinolone and clobetasol cream, are used on other areas of the body. To help increase absorption and maximize effectiveness of topical steroids, patients are instructed to apply a topical emollient, such as Aquaphor, 30 minutes following steroid application. In addition, the skin can be covered with warm wet towels as an occlusive measure ("wet wrap"). For more intense and resistant rashes, topical tacrolimus may be used.

Table 3
Topical agents for acute GVHD

Medication	Strength (%)	Dose	Location	Comments
Hydrocortisone	1 (low potency)	Apply to affected area twice daily	Face, axilla, groin	Long-term use acceptable
Desonide	0.05 (mild potency)	Apply to affected area twice daily	Face, axilla, groin	—
Triamcinolone	0.1 (moderate potency)	Apply to affected area twice daily	Body	Avoid face, axilla, and groin
Clobetasol (Temovate)	0.05 (high potency)	Apply to affected area twice daily	Limit to active area	Avoid face, axilla, and groin; limit use to 2 wk at a time
Fluocinonide (Lidex)	0.05 (high potency)	Apply to affected area twice daily	Scalp	Limit use to 2 wk at a time
Tacrolimus (Protopic)	0.1	Apply to affected area twice daily	—	—

When cutaneous GVHD involvement is grade II or higher, systemic therapy is initiated. Corticosteroids have remained the first-line therapy for aGVHD for decades. Prior studies have evaluated initial dosing of steroids (1 mg/kg/day vs 2 mg/kg/day) and concluded that initial treatment with low-dose glucocorticoids for patients with grades I to II GVHD did not compromise disease control or mortality and was associated with decreased toxicity.[20] For patients with cutaneous aGVHD receiving prednisone, overall improvement was observed at Day 28 of treatment in 55% of patients, with durable ($\geq$28 days) complete response observed in 35% and partial response observed in 20% of patients.[21] Once GVHD manifestations have resolved, prednisone is tapered by 0.2 mg/kg/day every 3 to 5 days with close monitoring. The taper schedules provided in multicenter trials for aGVHD (ie, Blood and Marrow Transplant Clinical Trials Network 0302 or 0802) reflect current practice and are appropriate guidelines.[22]

GI aGVHD is a complicated and serious entity in the transplant patient. It is distinguished between upper and lower GI involvement. Treatment of the upper GI aGVHD entails nonabsorbable steroids, such as budesonide (Entocort), in addition to systemic steroids (eg, prednisone). Oral nonabsorbable steroids, such as budesonide and beclomethasone, can increase response rates and allow for lower doses of systemic steroids.[23] Lower GI aGVHD also requires systemic steroids. These patients should be evaluated by a nutritionist because they can become malnourished and develop abnormalities in magnesium, zinc, vitamin B_{12}, and vitamin D.[24] Patients with diarrhea exceeding 500 mL/day should be considered for total parenteral nutrition, with gradual introduction of oral intake once the diarrhea decreases to less than 500 mL/day. Treatment of liver aGVHD also involves initial therapy with high-dose systemic steroids.

Patients who fail to respond to systemic steroids within 7 days or display progression within 72 hours are considered to be steroid-refractory. These patients are considered to be glucocorticoid resistant and require second-line therapy. A wide range of investigational treatments are used, but there is no standardization. The following agents are suggested for use in the second-line treatment of steroid-refractory aGVHD: extracorporeal photopheresis, anti–tumor necrosis factor-α antibodies, mammalian target of rapamycin inhibitors, mycophenolate mofetil, and interleukin-2 receptor antibodies (**Table 4**).[19]

Management of Chronic Graft-Versus-Host Disease

Initial therapy for cGVHD depends on extent of organ involvement (see **Table 2**). Indications for systemic therapy are involvement of three or more organs,[13] any single organ with severity score greater than 2,[13] persistent thrombocytopenia (platelet count <100,000/μL),[25,26] and cGVHD that has evolved from aGVHD.[27]

Similar to aGVHD, corticosteroids remain the mainstay of initial treatment of cGVHD. Steroids are generally initiated at a dose of 1 mg/kg/day.[28] Response to steroids is assessed approximately 2 weeks after initiating therapy with the intent to taper by 25% every week. Once symptoms have resolved, one should continue a slow taper until steroids are completely discontinued.

Patients who develop cGVHD while receiving systemic glucocorticoids are treated with additional agents for resistant disease (**Table 5**). The host of second-line agents in GVHD is primarily investigational. Therapies considered in the setting of steroid-refractory cGVHD include extracorporeal photopheresis, sirolimus, rituximab, tyrosine kinase inhibitors, interleukin-2, and methoxsalen and ultraviolet A radiation.[29–35]

There are some notable adjunctive treatment options specific to each organ site worth mentioning.[36] For GVHD of the skin, emollients are frequently used, and antihistamines may also be used for patients with pruritus. Topical steroids and topical

Table 4
Second-line therapy for acute GVHD

Medication	Strength	Dose
Extracorporeal photopheresis	Performed twice weekly and tapered based on response	Requires Hickman catheter Particularly effective in cutaneous, hepatic, and pulmonary GVHD
Mycophenolate mofetil (Cellcept)	1 g po bid	May cause nausea or diarrhea
Rituximab (Rituxan)	375 mg/m^2 IV × 4 weekly doses	Benefits cutaneous GVHD; can cause B-cell aplasia
Pentostatin (Nipent)	1.5 mg/m^2 IV Day 1, 2, 3 and 15, 16, 17 OR 4 mg/m^2 IV Day 1 and 15	Major risk of infection and cytopenias
Etanercept (Enbrel)	0.4 mg/kg (max: 25 mg) sq twice weekly for up to 8 weeks	—
Sirolimus	On azole: 0.2–0.4 mg/d No azole: 1–4 mg/d	Target trough level is 7–10 ng/mL; monitor levels weekly; can cause hyperlipidemia; should be managed by a clinician experienced with this medication

Abbreviations: IV, intravenous; SQ, subcutaneous.

Table 5
Second-line therapy for chronic GVHD

Treatment	Dose	Comments
Extracorporeal photopheresis	Performed twice weekly and tapered based on response	Requires Hickman catheter Particularly effective in cutaneous, hepatic, and pulmonary GVHD
Rituximab	375 mg/m^2 IV × 4 weekly doses	Benefits cutaneous GVHD
Sirolimus	On azole: 0.2–0.4 mg/d No azole: 1–4 mg/d	Target trough level is 7–10 ng/mL; monitor levels weekly; can cause hyperlipidemia; should be manage by clinician experienced with this medication
Imatinib (Gleevec)	Initial: 100–200 mg/d po (max: 400 mg/d)	Best for refractory sclerotic GVHD May cause fluid retention and myelosuppression (monitor counts)
Pentostatin	1.5 mg/m^2 IV Day 1, 2, 3 and 15, 16, 17 OR 4 mg/m^2 IV Day 1 and 15	Major risk of infection and cytopenias
Interleukin-2 (Proleukin)	1 million IU/m^2 sq daily (8 wk on; 4 wk off)	First exclude TTP/TMA/HUS Check CBC, Cr 3–4 d after starting Only stable for 14 d at a time if patient is self-administering (keep refrigerated)

Abbreviations: CBC, complete blood count; Cr, creatinine; HUS, hemolytic uremic syndrome; IV, intravenous; SQ, subcutaneous; TMA, thrombotic microangiopathy; TTP, thrombotic thrombocytopenic purpura.

tacrolimus may be helpful when used sparingly, and close follow-up with a dermatologist can also be beneficial. Oral cGVHD symptoms can benefit from topical steroid mouthwashes or clobetasol used sparingly. Preservative-free artificial tears, lacrimal duct plugs, and steroid drops can alleviate severe ocular dryness, and referral to an ophthalmologist who specializes in ocular cGVHD may be necessary. Vaginal dryness, atrophy, and stenosis is seen in vaginal cGVHD and warrants prompt evaluation by a gynecologist for consideration of lubricants, topical estrogens, or vaginal dilators.[37] Untreated vaginal GVHD can progress to agglutination of the vaginal wall, causing dyspareunia and significant impairment on quality of life. Patients with lung involvement are often started on inhaled corticosteroids, such as fluticasone (Flovent), 220 µg twice daily, to maximize lung function. Pulmonary rehabilitation can also be beneficial in patients whose activities of daily living are severely impacted.[38] Patients who have fascial involvement may have limitation in range of motion with joint contractures.[39] These patients should undergo a formal physical therapy evaluation with therapeutic emphasis on the affected limbs. In addition, all patients with GVHD treated with steroids should undergo aggressive muscle strengthening exercises to regain muscle mass lost from chronic steroid use. Adjunctive therapies and prompt referral are instrumental in the recovery of patients suffering from cGVHD.

Toxicities Related to Immunosuppressive Agents

The treatments used for managing acute and cGVHD can have tremendous negative consequences if not carefully managed by an experienced clinician. It is of utmost importance to have familiarity with the treatment modality to reduce toxicity of a particular medication. Side effects of tacrolimus include renal insufficiency and magnesium wasting. Therefore, patients may require intravenous fluids and high doses of oral magnesium supplementation. Toxicities associated with supratherapeutic tacrolimus levels (ie, >10 ng/mL) include tremor, headache, hypertension, and nephrotoxicity. Tacrolimus has an elimination half-life of approximately 12 hours. Similarly, sirolimus requires close monitoring, particularly given its long half-life of approximately 62 hours. Toxicities associated with sirolimus include headache, hypertension, hyperlipidemia, and thrombotic thrombocytopenic purpura. It is imperative that providers monitor fasting serum triglyceride levels periodically while on sirolimus and treat hypertriglyceridemia accordingly. Providers must also be cautious when prescribing new medications to avoid potentially harmful drug interactions with calcineurin inhibitors because they are metabolized by hepatic cytochrome P-450 enzymes.

COMPLICATIONS OF GRAFT-VERSUS-HOST DISEASE MANAGEMENT

Sequelae of cGVHD include numerous deleterious effects, such as functional limitations, issues with self-image, and organ failure. Moreover, treatment of cGVHD requires prolonged immunosuppressive regimens, such as corticosteroids and tacrolimus, which can result in numerous complications including avascular necrosis (AVN), secondary malignancies, infections, and adrenal insufficiency. Although the patient's disease may be cured by allo-HSCT, complications from GVHD and immunosuppressive regimens largely contribute to posttransplant morbidity and can profoundly diminish quality of life.

Infection Caused by Immune Dysregulation

Allo-HSCT recipients often receive myeloablative chemotherapy regimens before stem cell infusion to eradicate disease and deplete the recipient's immune system to enable engraftment of donor cells. Immune reconstitution is a timely process and immune system functionality is impaired by cGVHD and the immunosuppressive agents used for treatment. While immune suppressed, patients are susceptible to numerous infections. Encapsulated organisms (*Streptococcus pneumoniae, Haemophilus influenzae,* and *Neisseria meningitidis*) are a common source of infection in patients with cGVHD treated with corticosteroids. Patients are also at risk for opportunistic infection, such as *Pneumocystis* pneumonia and invasive fungal infections (eg, mucormycosis and aspergillosis). Furthermore, viral infections, such as community-acquired respiratory viruses, varicella zoster, or cytomegalovirus reactivation, are common in the transplant recipient. Because myeloablative chemotherapy depletes the patient's lymphocytes, immune memory is rapidly lost after transplant. Therefore, the Centers for Disease Control and Prevention recommends initiating inactivated vaccines approximately 6 months posttransplant for allo-HSCT and auto-HSCT recipients (**Table 6**).[40] Furthermore, live-attenuated viruses, such as measles/mumps/rubella and varicella vaccines, cannot be administered until at least 2 years posttransplant and once a patient is off immune suppression because of increased risk of contracting disease.[40] In summary, patients on immune suppression should remain on antimicrobial prophylaxis, be closely monitored for infectious diseases, minimize infectious exposure, and be up to date on vaccinations.

Endocrinopathies

Transplant chemotherapy and radiation causes significant hormonal dysregulation. For example, 95% of posttransplant females develop hypergonadotropic hypogonadism and ovarian insufficiency resulting in early menopause and secondary amenorrhea, which can lead to early osteoporosis.[41] Semen analysis in posttransplant males reveals azoospermia, and patients have increased follicular-stimulating hormone levels suggestive of spermatogenesis dysfunction.[41] Additionally, the management of cGVHD often requires prolonged corticosteroids, and tapering can induce secondary adrenal

Table 6
CDC recommendations for posttransplant vaccinations

Vaccine	Months Posttransplant				
	6	9	12	18	24+
Inactivated polio	X	X	X		
DTaP	X	X	X		
Haemophilus influenzae type b	X	X	X		
Hepatitis B[a]	X	X	X		
Pneumococcal conjugate (PCV13)	X	X	X	X	
Inactivated influenza[b]	X				
MMR					X
Varicella					X

Auto-HSCT and allo-HSCT recipients are recommended to have immunizations posttransplant because of loss of immune memory with myeloblative chemotherapy. Live virus vaccines (ie, MMR and varicella) cannot be administered until at least 24 months posttransplant and once patient is off immunosuppression for at least 3 months. Optional vaccinations include human papilloma virus, meningococcal, and hepatitis A (refer to CDC guidelines).

Abbreviations: CDC, Centers for Disease Control and Prevention; DTaP, full dose diphtheria/tetanus/acellular pertussis; MMR, measles/mumps/rubella.

[a] For seropositive hepatitis B donor/recipients, refer to CDC guidelines and consider early vaccination and nucleoside analogue.

[b] Inactivated influenza is to be given at 6 months posttransplant and annually for the remainder of the patient's life.

insufficiency caused by adrenocorticotropic hormone suppression. Patients undergoing a steroid taper with fatigue, weakness, or weight loss should undergo proper work-up including morning serum cortisol level and cosyntropin stimulation testing to determine if hydrocortisone replacement is indicated.

Avascular Necrosis

AVN is a major complication of allo-HSCT. The cause of AVN in allo-HSCT recipients is controversial; however, studies have repeatedly shown an increased propensity for developing AVN in patients with GVHD who receive steroid therapy.[42–44] AVN can affect any joint, although the femoral head is most commonly involved. Patients often report joint pain or have nontraumatic fractures, and diagnosis is confirmed with plain radiographs. AVN is quite debilitating and requires prompt referral to an orthopedist to consider surgical intervention.

Secondary Malignancy

Conditioning regimens for allo-HSCT include combinations of various chemotherapeutic agents with or without total body irradiation. Exposure to these mutagenic agents and prolonged immune suppression can lead to the development of secondary malignancies, such as therapy-related myelodysplastic syndrome/acute myeloid leukemia, melanoma, basal cell carcinoma, and head and neck cancers. The estimated cumulative 10-year risk of developing a secondary cancer after allo-HSCT is approximately 9%.[45] In general, risk factors of secondary malignancies include sun exposure and tobacco use, and patients should be adequately counseled. Patients with allo-HSCT should be diligently screened for secondary malignancies indefinitely.

SUMMARY

GVHD is a pleomorphic, multisystem disease that is a common complication of allo-HSCT. The clinical presentation is variable and requires prompt diagnosis, treatment, and proper referral. Furthermore, long-term complications of GVHD and its management include infectious risk, endocrinopathies, treatment toxicities, AVN, and secondary malignancies. Allo-HSCT recipients should be thoroughly screened for GVHD and long-term complications at every clinic visit, and concerning findings should always be relayed to the transplant physician and team for further evaluation and management of this complex disease.

REFERENCES

1. Gratwohl PA, Pasquini MC, Aljurf PM, et al. One million haemopoietic stem-cell transplants: a retrospective observational study. Lancet Haematol 2015;2:91–100.
2. Barnes DWH, Corp MJ, Loutit JF, et al. Treatment of murine leukaemia with x-rays and homologous bone marrow. Br Med J 1956;2:626–7.
3. Welniak LA, Blazar BR, Murphy WJ. Immunobiology of allogeneic hematopoietic stem cell transplantation. Annu Rev Immunol 2007;25:139–70.
4. Billingham RE. The biology of graft-versus-host reactions. Harvey Lect 1966–1967;62:21–78.
5. Ferrara JLM, Levine JE, Reddy P, et al. Graft-versus-host disease. Lancet 2009; 273:1550–61.
6. Korngold R, Sprent J. T cell subsets and graft-versus-host disease. Transplantation 1987;44(3):335–9.

7. Flowers ME, Inamoto Y, Carpenter PA, et al. Comparative analysis of risk factors for acute graft-versus-host disease and for chronic graft-versus-host disease according to National Institutes of Health consensus criteria. Blood 2011;117:3214–9.

8. Jagasia M, Arora M, Flowers ME, et al. Risk factors for acute GVHD and survival after hematopoietic cell transplantation. Blood 2012;119:296–307.

9. Rocha V, Locatelli F. Searching for alternative hematopoietic stem cell donors for pediatric patients. Bone Marrow Transplant 2008;41:207–14.

10. Glucksberg H, Storb R, Fefer A, et al. Clinical manifestations of graft-versus-host disease in human recipients of marrow from HLA-matched sibling donors. Transplantation 1974;18(4):295–304.

11. Przepiorka D, Weisdorf D, Martin P, et al. 1994 consensus conference on acute GVHD grading. Bone Marrow Transplant 1995;15(6):825–8.

12. Shulman HM, Sullivan KM, Weiden PL, et al. Chronic graft-versus-host syndrome in man. A long-term clinicopathologic study of 20 Seattle patients. Am J Med 1980;69(2):204–17.

13. Filipovich AH, Weisdorf D, Pavletic S, et al. National Institutes of Health consensus development project on criteria for clinical trials in chronic graft-versus-host disease: I. Diagnosis and staging working group report. Biol Blood Marrow Transplant 2005;11:945–56.

14. Jagasia MH, Greinix HT, Arora M, et al. National Institutes of Health consensus development project on criteria for clinical trials in chronic graft-versus-host disease: I. The 2014 Diagnosis and Staging Working Group report. Biol Blood Marrow Transplant 2015;21(3):389–401.

15. Cahn JY, Klein JP, Lee SJ, et al. Prospective evaluation of 2 acute graft-versus-host (GVHD) grading systems: a joint Société Française de Greffe de Moëlle et Thérapie Cellulaire (SFGM-TC), Dana Farber Cancer Institute (DFCI), and International Bone Marrow Transplant Registry (IBMTR) prospective study. Blood 2005;106:1495–500.

16. Lee SJ, Klein JP, Barrett AJ, et al. Severity of chronic graft-versus-host disease: association with treatment-related mortality and relapse. Blood 2002;100:406–14.

17. Erard V, Chien JW, Kim HW, et al. Airflow decline after myeloablative allogeneic hematopoietic cell transplantation: the role of community respiratory viruses. J Infect Dis 2006;193:1619–25.

18. Jacobsohn DA, Vogelsang GB. Acute graft versus host disease. Orphanet J Rare Dis 2007;2:35.

19. Dignan FL, Clark A, Amrolia P, et al. Diagnosis and management of acute graft-versus-host disease. Br J Haematol 2012;158:30.

20. Mielcarek M, Storer BE, Boeckh M, et al. Initial therapy of acute graft-versus-host disease with low-dose prednisone does not compromise patient outcomes. Blood 2009;113:2888.

21. MacMillan ML, Weisdorf DJ, Wagner JE, et al. Response of 443 patients to steroids as primary therapy for acute graft-versus-host disease: comparison of grading systems. Biol Blood Marrow Transplant 2002;8:387.

22. Martin PJ, Rizzo JD, Wingard JR, et al. First- and second-line systemic treatment of acute graft-versus-host disease: recommendations of the American Society of Blood and Marrow Transplantation. Biol Blood Marrow Transplant 2012;18:1150.

23. Ibrahim RB, Abidi MH, Cronin SM, et al. Nonabsorbable corticosteroids use in the treatment of gastrointestinal graft-versus-host disease. Biol Blood Marrow Transplant 2009;15:395.

24. van der Meij BS, de Graaf P, Wierdsma NJ, et al. Nutritional support in patients with GVHD of the digestive tract: state of the art. Bone Marrow Transplant 2013;48:474.

25. Sullivan KM, Witherspoon RP, Storb R, et al. Prednisone and azathioprine compared with prednisone and placebo for treatment of chronic graft-v-host disease: prognostic influence of prolonged thrombocytopenia after allogeneic marrow transplantation. Blood 1988;72:546.

26. Sullivan KM, Witherspoon RP, Storb R, et al. Alternating-day cyclosporine and prednisone for treatment of high-risk chronic graft-v-host disease. Blood 1988; 72:555.

27. Wingard JR, Piantadosi S, Vogelsang GB, et al. Predictors of death from chronic graft-versus-host disease after bone marrow transplantation. Blood 1989;74: 1428.

28. Lee SJ, Vogelsang G, Flowers ME. Chronic graft-versus-host disease. Biol Blood Marrow Transplant 2003;9:215.

29. Dignan FL, Aguilar S, Scarisbrick JJ, et al. Impact of extracorporeal photopheresis on skin scores and quality of life in patients with steroid-refractory chronic GVHD. Bone Marrow Transplant 2014;49:704.

30. Couriel DR, Saliba R, Escalón MP, et al. Sirolimus in combination with tacrolimus and corticosteroids for the treatment of resistant chronic graft-versus-host disease. Br J Haematol 2005;130:409.

31. Alousi AM, Uberti J, Ratanatharathorn V. The role of B cell depleting therapy in graft versus host disease after allogeneic hematopoietic cell transplant. Leuk Lymphoma 2010;51:376.

32. Kim SJ, Lee JW, Jung CW, et al. Weekly rituximab followed by monthly rituximab treatment for steroid-refractory chronic graft-versus-host disease: results from a prospective, multicenter, phase II study. Haematologica 2010;95:1935.

33. Olivieri A, Cimminiello M, Corradini P, et al. Long-term outcome and prospective validation of NIH response criteria in 39 patients receiving imatinib for steroid-refractory chronic GVHD. Blood 2013;122:4111.

34. Koreth J, Matsuoka K, Kim HT, et al. Interleukin-2 and regulatory T cells in graft-versus-host disease. N Engl J Med 2011;365:2055.

35. Hymes SR, Morison WL, Farmer ER, et al. Methoxsalen and ultraviolet A radiation in treatment of chronic cutaneous graft-versus-host reaction. J Am Acad Dermatol 1985;12:30.

36. Dignan FL, Scarisbrick JJ, Cornish J, et al. Organ-specific management and supportive care in chronic graft-versus-host disease. Br J Haematol 2012;158:62–78.

37. Frey Tirri B, Häusermann P, Bertz H, et al. Clinical guidelines for gynecologic care after hematopoietic SCT. Report from the international consensus project on clinical practice in chronic GVHD. Bone Marrow Transplant 2015;50:3.

38. Hildebrandt GC, Fazekas T, Lawitschka A, et al. Diagnosis and treatment of pulmonary chronic GVHD: report from the consensus conference on clinical practice in chronic GVHD. Bone Marrow Transplant 2011;46:1283.

39. Marks C, Stadler M, Häusermann P, et al. German-Austrian-Swiss Consensus Conference on clinical practice in chronic graft-versus-host disease (GVHD): guidance for supportive therapy of chronic cutaneous and musculoskeletal GVHD. Br J Dermatol 2011;165:18.

40. Kroger AT, Sumaya CV, Pickering LK, et al. Centers for Disease Control and Prevention. General recommendations on immunization: recommendations of the advisory committee on immunization practices. MMWR Recomm Rep 2011; 60(2):1–60.

41. Tauchmanovà L, Selleri C, De Rosa G, et al. High prevalence of endocrine dysfunction in long-term survivors after allogeneic bone marrow transplantation for hematologic disease. Cancer 2002;95:1076–84.

42. Stern JM, Sullivan KM, Ott SM, et al. Bone density loss after allogeneic hematopoietic stem cell transplantation: a prospective study. Biol Blood Marrow Transplant 2001;7:257–64.

43. Torii Y, Hasegawa Y, Kubo T, et al. Osteonecrosis of the femoral head after allogeneic bone marrow transplantation. Clin Orthop Relat Res 2001;(382):124–32.

44. Tauchmanovà L, De Rosa G, Serio B, et al. Avascular necrosis in long-term survivors after allogeneic or autologous stem cell transplantation. Cancer 2003;97:2453–61.

45. Lowsky R, Lipton J, Fyles G, et al. Secondary malignancies after bone marrow transplantation in adults. J Clin Oncol 1994;12:2187–92.

New Pharmaceutical Agents in Oncology

Christine Cambareri, PharmD, BCPS, BCOP[a], Carmen F. Nobre, PharmD, BCOP[b],*,
Laura A. Tuttle, PharmD, BCOP[b]

KEYWORDS

- Monoclonal antibody • Tyrosine kinase inhibitors • Oral chemotherapy
- Targeted therapy • Immunotherapy • 2015

KEY POINTS

- Targeted therapy against overexpressed and mutated proteins and receptors is becoming a cornerstone of oncology care.
- Immunotherapy in oncology provides a novel therapeutic approach against cancer, as well as a side effect profile distinct from conventional cytotoxic chemotherapy.
- Targeted small-molecule drugs are a chief focus for drug development in oncology because of their involvement in growth factor signaling. Their convenience and activity against cancer cells make them desirable treatment options.

Oncology is constantly changing with the development of new therapies. In the last 5 years, more than 50 new oncologic indications and/or drugs have received US Food and Drug Administration (FDA) approval. This article focuses on agents approved in 2015.

MONOCLONAL ANTIBODIES

The use of monoclonal antibody (mAb) treatment of cancer has been established as one of the most successful treatment strategies within oncology in the past 30 years.[1] The advances within this realm of targeted therapy since inception in 1975 and first approval of an oncologic monoclonal antibody in 1997 with rituximab (Rituxan) have been unparalleled. At present there are more than 20 mAbs approved for the treatment of cancer, with 13 FDA approvals and expansion of indications occurring in the year 2015 alone.[2] Identification of overexpressed, selectively expressed, or mutated

Disclosure: The authors have nothing to disclose.
[a] Perelman Center for Advanced Medicine, Abramson Cancer Center, Hospital of the University of Pennsylvania, West Pavilion, 3400 Civic Center Boulevard, Philadelphia, PA 19104, USA;
[b] Department of Pharmacy, Smilow Cancer Hospital at Yale New Haven, 20 York Street, New Haven, CT 06510, USA
* Corresponding author.
E-mail address: Carmen.Nobre@ynhh.org

targets on cell surfaces of cancer cells has made the use of mAbs possible in oncology.[3]

Advancements in the production of mAbs have also contributed heavily to the continued success of this therapeutic modality. The earliest mAb treatments were entirely murine based, therefore completely foreign to humans with serious immune-mediated reaction concerns. Engineering practices have changed to minimize this concern with the development of chimeric antibodies with fusion of mouse and human domains (**Fig. 1**).[4–8]

The variety of mechanisms and targets by which mAbs exert their anticancer effects enable these agents to be used in combination with cytotoxic therapies and with each other to have their maximal effects. These various mechanisms of action include direct cell killing, immune-mediated cell killing, and specific effects on tumor vasculature and stroma (as described in **Box 1**). Antibody drug conjugates (ADC) are mAbs covalently linked to cytotoxic molecules and are used to deliver the cytotoxic therapy to the target cells.

Newly approved mAbs and expanded indications in the year 2015 are discussed here.

ANTI-CD30

The target CD30 is a transmembrane receptor protein that is primarily expressed on Reed-Sternberg cells characteristic of Hodgkin lymphoma (HL) and systemic anaplastic large cell lymphoma (sALCL) cells.[9] CD30 expression is associated with T-cell activation, which drives malignant cellular growth. Brentuximab vedotin (Adcetris) offers overall response rates (ORR) of greater than 70% in patients with relapsed HL in patients who are not candidates for transplant, relapsed HL after an autologous stem cell transplant (SCT), and relapsed sALCL (**Table 1**).[10] In August of 2015, brentuximab also received approval to be given as consolidation therapy after autologous SCT for patients who are at high risk of relapse or progression. Dosing and administration specifics are detailed in **Box 2**.

Brentuximab is an ADC composed of a chimeric CD30 immunoglobulin mAb connected to a microtubule disrupting agent, known as monomethyl auristain E (MMAE). When the ADC binds to CD30 on the cell surface, it is internalized and cleaved, unleashing MMAE to disrupt the cell's microtubule network and causing apoptosis of the CD30-expressing tumor cell.

The adverse drug events (ADEs) occurring in more than 20% of patients are neutropenia, peripheral neuropathy, fatigue, nausea, anemia, upper respiratory tract

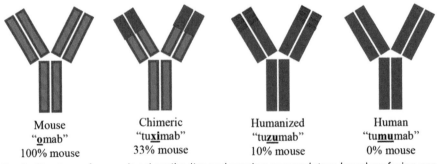

Mouse	Chimeric	Humanized	Human
"omab"	"tuximab"	"tuzumab"	"tumumab"
100% mouse	33% mouse	10% mouse	0% mouse

Fig. 1. Structure of monoclonal antibodies and naming nomenclature based on fusion protein types.

Box 1
Monoclonal antibody mechanisms of kill

Direct cell killing

• Apoptosis caused by inhibited signaling and proliferation from receptor blockade

• Apoptosis caused by cell receptor agonist activity

• Signal abrogation from cell enzyme surface neutralization

• Delivery of drug from a conjugated drug antibody, radiation, or other cytotoxic agent

Immune-mediated cell killing

• Induction of phagocytosis

• Complement activation

• Antibody-dependent cell-mediated cytotoxicity

• Regulation of T-cell function

Specific effects on tumor vasculature and stroma

• Antagonism of the vessel receptor

• Stromal cell inhibition

• Delivery of drug from a conjugated drug antibody

---

infection, and diarrhea.[11] The incidence of neuropathy was particularly high at 54% in the clinical trial experiences and warrants dose reductions in patients during therapy.[10]

As a chimeric antibody, brentuximab carries a risk for infusion reactions. Although routine premedication is not recommended, patients experiencing an infusion-related reaction should receive premedication with acetaminophen, an antihistamine, and a corticosteroid before all subsequent infusions. This agent carries a black box warning for progressive multifocal leukoencephalopathy (PML), a demyelinating encephalopathy. Because the PML is T-cell driven, reactivation of the opportunistic JC virus often happens sooner than with anti-CD20 therapy, which is B-cell driven.[12]

Unlike other mAb therapies, brentuximab has a potential for drug interactions because of the MMAE component.[13] Strong cytochrome P (CYP) 3A4 enzyme inhibitors and inducers and p-glycoprotein inhibitors should be avoided during brentuximab therapy inhibitors (see Supplemental Material for discussion of drug-drug interactions).

ANTI-CD38

Multiple myeloma (MM) cells highly and homogeneously express the transmembrane glycoprotein CD38. The role of this protein in MM cells is regulation of calcium flux, signal transduction, and cell perpetuity. The amount of CD38 expressed on normal lymphoid and myeloid cells and some tissues of nonhematopoietic origin is low, making CD38 an attractive target for MM treatment. The first anti-CD38 antibody, daratumumab (Darzalex), was approved in November of 2015. Daratumumab was granted accelerated approval based on response rates of 29.2% and 36% in 2 open-label trials in relapsed or refractory disease in patients who received at least 2 prior therapies.[14,15] Dosing and administration specifics are detailed in **Box 3**.

The infusion titration is an integral part of administration of this therapy because of the 46% incidence of infusion reactions during clinical trials. Infusion reactions often occur during the first infusion or the first 4 hours after the infusion is complete. If

Table 1
Summary of clinical trials of oncology monoclonal antibody therapy

Drug	Study Design	Population	Results

Brentuximab (Adcetris)	Open label, single arm, (n = 102)	R/R HL after auto	• CR: 32% (95% CI: 23, 42)
			  ○ Median DOR: 20.5 mo
			• PR: 40% (95% CI: 32, 29)
			  ○ Median DOR: 3.5 mo
			• ORR: 73% (95% CI: 65, 83)
			  ○ Median DOR: 6.7 mo

	Open label, single arm, (n = 58)	R/R sALCL	• CR: 57% (95% CI: 44, 70)
			  ○ Median DOR: 13.2 mo
			• PR: 29% (95% CI: 18, 41)
			  ○ Median DOR: 2.1 mo
			• ORR: 86% (95% CI: 77, 95)
			  ○ Median DOR: 12.6 mo

	Randomized, double-blind RCT comparing B with PCB, (n = 329)	High-risk HL after auto HSCT	• mPFS: 42.9 vs 24.1 mo favoring B ○ HR = 0.57 (0.40, 0.81), P = .001
Daratumumab (Darzalex)	Open-label, phase II trial, (n = 106)	R/R MM with 3 prior therapies	• ORR: 29.2% • Median time to response: 1 mo • Median DOR: 7.4 mo
	Open-label, dose escalation trial, (n = 72)	R/R MM with 2 prior therapies	• ORR: 36% • Median time to response: 1 mo • Median DOR: 6.9 mo • OS rate at 12 mo: 77%

Agent	Trial	Population	Outcomes

Ramucirumab (Cyramza)	Double-blind RCT comparing R vs PCB, (n = 355)	Advanced or metastatic gastric cancer failing platinum or 5-FU therapy	• OS: 5.2 vs 3.8 mo favoring R
			  ○ HR: 0.78 (95% CI: 0.60, 0.998), $P = .047$
			• PFS: 2.1 vs 1.3 mo favoring R
			  ○ HR: 0.48 (95% CI: 0.38, 0.62), $P<.001$

	Double blind RCT comparing R + paclitaxel (T) vs PCB + T, (n = 665)		• OS: 9.6 vs 7.4 mo favoring R + T
			  ○ HR: 0.81 (95% CI: 0.68, 0.96), $P = .017$
			• PFS: 4.4 vs 2.9 mo favoring (R + T)
			  ○ HR: 0.64 (95% CI: 0.54, 0.75), $P<.001$
			• ORR: 28% vs 16% favoring (R + T)
			  ○ $P<.001$

	Double-blind RCT comparing R + D vs PCB + D, (n = 1253)	Advanced or metastatic NSCLC failing platinum therapy	• OS: 10.5 vs 9.1 mo favoring (R + D)
			  ○ HR: 0.86 (95% CI: 0.75, 0.98), $P = .024$
			• PFS: 4.5 vs 3.0 mo favoring (R + D)
			  ○ HR: 0.76 (95% CI: 0.68, 0.86), $P<.001$
			• ORR: 23% vs 14% favoring (R + D)
			  ○ $P<.001$

	Double-blind RCT comparing R + FOLFIRI vs PCB + FOLFIRI, (n = 1072)	mCRC failing platinum, bevacizumab + 5-FU	• OS: 13.3 vs 11.7 mo favoring (R + FOLFIRI)
			  ○ HR: 0.85 (95% CI: 0.73, 0.98), $P = .023$
			• PFS: 5.7 vs 4.5 mo favoring (R + FOLFIRI)
			  ○ HR: 0.79 (95% CI: 0.7, 0.90), $P<.001$

Necitumumab (Portrazza)	SQUIRE Trial: Open-label, phase 3, RCT comparing necitumumab, gemcitabine, cisplatin (NGC) vs GC, (n = 1093)	Previously untreated stage IV squamous NSCLC	• OS: 11.5 vs 9.9 mo favoring (NGC)
			  ○ HR: 0.84 (95% CI: 0.74–0.96), $P = .01$
			• mPFS: 5.7 vs 5.5 mo favoring (NGC)
			  ○ HR: 0.85 (95% CI: 0.74–0.98), $P = .02$
			• mTTF: 4.3 vs 3.6 mo favoring (NGC)
			• ORR: 31% vs 29% favoring (NGC)

Elotuzumab (Empliciti)	ELOQUENT-2: Phase 3, RCT comparing elotuzumab + lenalidomide + dexamethasone (ERd) or (Rd), (n = 646)	R/R MM	• PFS 1 y with ERd: 68% vs 57% with Rd
			• PFS 2 y with ERd:41% vs 27% with Rd
			• mPFS: 19.4 vs 14.9 mo favoring ERd
			  ○ ($P<.001$)
			• ORR: 79% vs 66% favoring ERd
			  ○ ($P<.001$)
			• The ERd regimen resulted in a 30% reduction in the risk of disease progression or death compared with Rd alone
			  ○ HR 0.70 (95% CI: 0.57, 0.85), $P = .0004$

(continued on next page)

Table 1
(continued)

Drug	Study Design	Population	Results

Ipilimumab (Yervoy)	Double-blind RCT comparing I vs immune vaccine plus (I + V) vs V, (n = 676)	Unresectable or metastatic melanoma	• mOS = 10.1 vs 10 vs 6.4 mo for I vs (I + V) vs (V).
			  ○ IV HR 0.68, (95% CI: 0.55, 0.85), P = .0004
			  ○ I HR 0.66, (95% CI: 0.51, 0.87), P = .0026

	RCT comparing I vs placebo PCB, (n = 951)	Resectable melanoma	• RFS: 26 vs 17 mo favoring I ○ HR: 0.75 (95% CI: 0.64, 0.90), P<.002

Pembrolizumab (Keytruda)	Open-label RCT comparing pembrolizumab at 10 mg/kg every 2 wk (P2) vs 10 mg/kg every 3 wk (P3) vs I, (n = 834)	Unresectable or metastatic melanoma	• Death: 33% vs 30% vs 40% for (P3, P2, I)
			  ○ (P2) HR: 0.63 (95% CI: 0.47, 0.83), P<.001
			• PFS: 4.1 vs 5.5 vs 2.8 mo favoring P2
			  ○ (P2) HR: 0.58 (95% CI: 0.46, 0.72), P<.001
			• ORR: 33% vs 34% vs 12% favoring P3 and P2

	RCT comparing pembrolizumab 2 mg/kg (2P) vs pembrolizumab 10 mg/kg (10P) vs C, (n = 540)	Unresectable or metastatic melanoma, refractory to ipilimumab	• PFS: 2.9 vs 2.9 vs 2.7 mo for (2P, 10P, C)
			  ○ 2P HR: 0.57 (95% CI: 0.45, 0.73), P<.001
			  ○ 10P HR: 0.5 (95% CI: 0.39, 0.64), P<.001
			• ORR: 21% vs 25% vs 4% favoring 2P and 10P

	Pembrolizumab 10 mg/kg every 2 or every 3 wk (P2, P3), n = 61	Metastatic NSCLC s/p platinum	• ORR: 41%
Nivolumab (Opdivo)	Open-label RCT comparing N vs chemotherapy (C), (n = 120)	R/R unresectable or metastatic melanoma	ORR: 32% (95% CI: 23, 41)

	Double-blind RCT comparing N vs D, (n = 418)	Untreated metastatic melanoma	• OS: not reached vs 10.8 mo favoring N
			  ○ HR: 0.42 (95% CI: 0.30, 0.60), P<.0001
			• PFS: 5.1 vs 2.2 mo favoring N
			  ○ HR: 0.43 (95% CI: 0.34, 0.56), P<.0001
			• ORR: 34% vs 9% favoring N

	Double-blind RCT comparing N + I vs N vs I, (n = 945)	Untreated metastatic melanoma	• PFS: 11.5 vs 6.9 vs 2.9 mo for (N + I, N, I) ○ NI HR: 0.42 (95% CI: 0.34,0.51), P<.0001 • ORR: 50% vs 40% vs 14% for (N + I, N, I)
	Open-label RCT comparing N with D (T), (n = 272)	Metastatic squamous NSCLC s/p progression	• OS: 9.2 vs 6.0 mo favoring N ○ HR: 0.59 (95% CI: 0.44, 0.79), P = .0025
	Open-label RCT comparing N vs E, (n = 821)	R/R advanced RCC	• OS: 25 vs 19.6 mo favoring N ○ HR: 0.73 (95% CI: 0.60, 0.89), P = .0018 • ORR: 21.5% vs 3.9% favoring N

Abbreviations: 5-FU, 5-fluorouracil; auto, autologous stem cell transplant; B, brentuximab; C, chemotherapy; CI, confidence interval; CR, complete response; D, dacarbazine; DOR, duration of response; E, everolimus; HR, hazard ratio; I, ipilimumab; mCRC, metastatic colorectal cancer; mPFS, median progression-free survival; N, nivolumab; NSCLC, non-small cell lung cancer; OS, overall survival; PCB; placebo; PR, partial response; R, ramucirumab; RCT, randomized controlled trial; R/R,

---

Box 2
Brentuximab (Adcetris)

- Dose: 1.8 mg/kg every 3 weeks until disease progression or unacceptable toxicity. Dose capped at 180 mg.

- Administration instructions: Given intravenously over 30 minutes.

- Renal impairment: no adjustment for mild to moderate impairment. Avoid in creatinine clearance (CrCl) less than 30 mL/min.

- Hepatic impairment: reduce to 1.2 mg/kg (maximum 120 mg) for Child-Pugh A. Avoid use in Child-Pugh B/C.

- Monitoring:
  - Complete blood count (CBC)
  - Peripheral neuropathy (reduce dose or discontinue therapy if severe)
  - Neurologic symptoms (black box warning: progressive multifocal leukoencephalopathy)
  - Infusion reactions
  - Electrolytes, including uric acid for tumor lysis

- Supportive care: acetaminophen, antihistamine, and corticosteroid as needed for infusion reaction management; antiemetics as needed

---

Box 3
Daratumumab (Darzalex)

- Dose: 16 mg/kg weekly during weeks 1 to 8, every 2 weeks during weeks 9 to 24, and every 4 weeks from week 25 onwards until disease progression.

- Administration instructions: the infusion is titrated during the first 3 infusions as follows:

	Dilution Volume (mL)	Initial Rate, First Hour (mL/h)	Rate Increments (mL/h)	Maximum Rate (mL/h)
First Infusion	1000	50	50 every hour	200
Second Infusion	500	50		
Subsequent Infusions	500	100		

Escalate during the second infusion only if there was not a grade 1 or greater infusion reaction during the first 3 hours of the first infusion. Escalate the third infusion only if the final infusion rate of greater than or equal to 100 mL/h is tolerated during the first 2 infusions.

- Renal impairment: no clinical studies done in patients with severe renal impairment.

- Hepatic impairment: no clinical studies done in patients with severe hepatic impairment.

- Monitoring:
  - CBC
  - Liver function tests (LFTs)
  - Infusion reactions

- Supportive care:
  - Acetaminophen, antihistamine, and corticosteroid as premedications 1 hour before infusion.
  - Additional steroids on the 2 days following the infusion to prevent delayed infusion reactions.
  - Antiviral prophylaxis against herpes zoster reactivation continued 3 months following therapy completion.
  - As-needed antiemetics.

patients react despite premedication, it is recommended to only resume the infusion at half the rate at which the reaction occurred and increase the rate as tolerated. If a patient has 3 occurrences of a grade 3 or greater infusion reaction despite the steps discussed earlier, permanently discontinue therapy.

In addition to infusion reactions, ADEs that occur at an incidence greater than 20% include fatigue, nausea, back pain, pyrexia, cough, upper respiratory tract infections, and bone marrow suppression. Daratumumab has the potential to interfere with cross matching and red blood cell antibody screening. Daratumumab binds to CD38 on red blood cells causing a positive Coombs test, therefore it is critical to type and screen patients before therapy initiation and inform the blood bank about the patient's therapy to ensure patients receive appropriately matched transfusions. This drug-mediated effect may persist for up to 6 months after the last infusion of daratumumab. Therapy can also interfere with the determination of complete response and possibly relapse from complete response in patients because of interference with assays used to monitor the M protein.

ANTI–VASCULAR ENDOTHELIAL GROWTH FACTOR

Vascular endothelial growth factor (VEGF) protein is involved in angiogenesis. The VEGF protein family secretes 6 proteins (VEGF-A, VEGF-B, VEGF-C, VEGF-D, VEGF-E, and placenta-induced growth factor), which bind to receptor tyrosine kinases that control signaling pathways needed to promote new blood vessel genesis. VEGF-A was found to be particularly important in tumor cell angiogenesis and became the target of the first anti-VEGF mAb, bevacizumab (Avastin), approved in 2004.[16]

Ten years later, another anti-VEGF mAb was approved: ramucirumab (Cyramza).[17] It is a fully human mAb, and targets more of the VEGF family by binding to VEGF receptor 2 and blocking the binding of the VEGF-A, VEGF-C, and VEGF-D. It offers increased overall survival (OS) and progression-free survival (PFS) in advanced or metastatic gastric cancer and non–small cell lung cancer (NSCLC). In April 2015 it was FDA approved for colorectal cancer after failure of first-line therapies.[18–21] The dosing and treatment interval among these indications vary (**Box 4**).

Both anti-VEGF mAbs carry black box warnings related to angiogenic ADE, including hemorrhage, hemoptysis, and gastrointestinal perforation.[22] In addition, because angiogenesis is integral to wound healing, anti-VEGF therapy should be discontinued at least 28 days before elective surgery and held until at least 28 days after surgery and until the wound is completely healed. Other angiogenic ADEs include hypertension, proteinuria, and arterial thromboembolic events. Therapy should be interrupted until hypertension is medically managed. If patients develop reversible posterior leukoencephalopathy syndrome caused by anti-VEGF-induced hypertension, permanently discontinue therapy. VEGF plays a role in normal glomerular development and preservation of glomerular filtration leading to a potential for development of proteinuria. If this develops, therapy should be interrupted. Ramucirumab carries a risk for infusion-related reactions; premedication recommendations can be found in **Box 4**.

ANTI–EPIDERMAL GROWTH FACTOR RECEPTOR

Growth factors, including the epidermal growth factor (EGF) family, play a role in unrestrained cellular promotion. EGF is a transmembrane protein that is part of the type I receptor tyrosine kinase family.[23] Ten different ligands can bind to each of these receptors, inducing receptor autophosphorylation to trigger intracellular pathways that result in cancer cell proliferation, inhibited apoptosis, metastasis formation, and tumor-induced neovascularization. Although EGF receptor (EGFR) is expressed in

---

Box 4
Ramucirumab (Cyramza)

• Doses:
  ○ Gastric cancer: 8 mg/kg intravenously every 2 weeks as a single agent or with paclitaxel
  ○ Non–small cell lung cancer: 10 mg/kg intravenously on day 1 of a 21-day cycle before docetaxel
  ○ Colorectal cancer: 8 mg/kg intravenously every 2 weeks, before FOLFIRI

• Administration instructions: given intravenously over 60 minutes. Administer through a separate line with a protein-sparing 0.22-μm filter and flush line with normal saline at the end of the infusion.

• Renal impairment: no clinical studies done in patients with severe renal impairment.

• Hepatic impairment: not applicable for mild/moderate hepatic impairment. Monitor liver function because clinical deterioration has been reported in patients with Child-Pugh B/C cirrhosis who received single-agent therapy.

• Monitoring:
  ○ CBC
  ○ LFTs
  ○ Infusion-related reactions
  ○ Blood pressure
  ○ Proteinuria
  ○ Arterial thromboembolic events

• Supportive care: premedication with an antihistamine for all patients, with or without corticosteroids and acetaminophen in patients who have experienced infusion reactions.

Abbreviation: FOLFIRI, FOL – Folinic acid (also called leucovorin, calcium folinate or FA) F – Fluorouracil (also called 5FU) IRI – Irinotecan (Campto).

---

many normal epithelial tissues, including the skin and hair follicles, there is also expression in head and neck, colon, and rectal cancers. The first EGFR antagonist approved was cetuximab (Erbitux) in 2004 for the treatment of squamous cell carcinoma of head and neck and K-RAS wild-type metastatic colorectal cancer. Because of its chimeric nature, therapy with cetuximab carries a black box warning for serious infusion reactions necessitating premedication.[24] Two additional human anti-EGFR mAb therapies with much lower incidences of infusion reactions have subsequently been approved: panitumumab (Vectibix) in 2006 and necitumumab (Portrazza) in 2015. Infusion reaction rates were less than 5%, thus neither agent requires upfront premedication against infusion reactions.

Necitumumab, the most recently approved anti-EGFR mAb (approved in November of 2015), is indicated in combination with gemcitabine and cisplatin as first-line treatment of metastatic squamous NSCLC.[25] Approval is based on combination therapy yielding a statistically significant longer OS, as shown in the SQUIRE trial (SQUamous NSCLC treatment with the Inhibitor of EGF REceptor) (see **Table 1**).[26] Trials were also done evaluating necitumumab in advanced nonsquamous NSCLC. The INSPIRE trial (Necitumumab plus pemetrexed and cisplatin as first-line therapy in patients with stage IV non-squamous non-small-cell lung cancer) found that the addition of necitumumab to cisplatin and pemetrexed in nonsquamous NSCLC showed more risk than benefit with an increase in treatment-related adverse events but similar OS, 11.3 months versus 11.5 months (hazard ratio [HR], 1.01; 95% confidence interval [CI], 0.84–1.21; P = .96).[27] Dosing and administration specifics are detailed in **Box 5**.

Significant side effects consistent with all 3 anti-EGFR mAbs include electrolyte depletion and dermatologic toxicities. Both cetuximab and necitumumab carry black

---

Box 5
Necitumumab (Portrazza)

- Dose: 800 mg on days 1 and 8 of each 3-week cycle.
- Administration instructions: given as an intravenous infusion over 60 minutes.
- Renal impairment: no clinical studies done in patients with severe renal impairment.
- Hepatic impairment: no clinical studies done in patients with severe hepatic impairment.
- Monitoring:
  ○ CBC
  ○ Electrolytes (especially magnesium, therapy carries a black box warning for hypomagnesemia)
  ○ Infusion-related reactions
  ○ Dermatologic toxicities
  ○ Venous and arterial thromboembolic events
- Supportive care:
  ○ Electrolyte repletion as needed.
  ○ Premedication with an antihistamine following a grade 1 to 2 infusion reaction.
  ○ Premedication with an antihistamine, acetaminophen, and steroids for a second grade 1 to 2 infusion reaction.

---

box warnings regarding cardiopulmonary arrest secondary to serum electrolyte imbalances, with necitumumab carrying a specific warning regarding hypomagnesemia because of an incidence of 83%. The mechanism behind the electrolyte imbalances is not fully understood. It has been postulated that there are EGFRs in the kidney, and inhibition affects the transient receptor potential cation channel, subfamily M, member 6 (TRPM6) in the distal collection duct, the main site of active renal magnesium reabsorption.[28] Strict monitoring and aggressive repletion of serum electrolytes is recommended during treatment and for up to 8 weeks after treatment in patients with EGFR antagonist therapy.

As mentioned previously, there is high expression of EGFR in the skin, especially the sebaceous epithelium, which includes the scalp, face, neck, chest, and upper back. Inhibition of EGFR causes class-wide cutaneous ADEs most commonly presenting as a papulopustular reaction.[29] Dermatologic toxicities are contained in warnings for all 3 drugs in this class, and are listed specifically as a black box warning for panitumumab with an incidence of 90%. Less frequent dermatologic presentations of EGFR inhibition include dry skin, pruritus, fissures, palmar-plantar rash, hyperkeratosis, telangiectasia, hyperpigmentation, blisters, mucositis, and pyogenic granuloma. Patients may also experience changes to their hair, including alopecia or trichomegaly of the eyelashes and paronychia of the nails. Symptoms usually develop within the first few weeks of treatment with erythema and edema on the skin, then a papulopustular eruption, followed by crusting that remains for the duration of the treatment and can be both painful and itchy.[30]

Skin toxicities tend to be more severe and widespread with mAb treatment compared with oral small-molecule tyrosine kinase inhibitors (TKIs) against EGFR. Because of the aggressiveness of this ADE, it is recommended that therapy be held and dose reduced proportionally to the severity of the skin reactions. Any patient who has persistent symptoms despite optimized supportive care, or dose delays or modifications should have therapy permanently discontinued. Supportive care measures that are often used for both prevention and treatment from the clinical practice guideline for EGFR-related toxicities supported by the Multinational Association of Supportive Care in Cancer (MASCC) are listed in **Box 6**.[31] Skin rash is often self-limited and resolves without

---

Box 6
Prevention and management of EGFR-induced skin toxicity

Prevention

- Topical: hydrocortisone 1% cream with moisturizer and sunscreen twice daily
- Systemic: minocycline 100 mg daily or doxycycline 100 mg twice daily

Treatment

- Topical: alclometasone 0.05% cream daily, fluocinonide 0.05% cream twice daily, or clindamycin 1% cream daily
- Systemic: doxycycline 100 mg twice daily, minocycline 100 mg daily, isotretinoin 20 to 30 mg/d

---

scarring through supportive care optimization and with discontinuation of EGFR antagonist therapy. However, the cutaneous reactions can negatively affect patient compliance and quality of life. All patients should be counseled on the risk of dermatologic toxicities when initiated on any drug within this class of therapy. There is also evidence that shows that tumor response and patient survival are improved in patients with a higher-severity rash from EGFR inhibitors. Cutaneous toxicity is currently considered as a surrogate marker for tumor response as well as OS.[32]

IMMUNOMODULATORY AGENTS

Blinatumomab (Blicynto) and elotuzumab (Empliciti) target proteins on B, T, and natural killer (NK) cells that are upregulated in some malignancies to stimulate the immune system to induce cell death. The first agent approved within this class was blinatumomab for the treatment of Philadelphia chromosome–negative relapsed refractory B-cell acute lymphoblastic leukemia in December of 2014.[33,34]

Elotuzumab, approved in November of 2015, targets SLAMF-7 on MM cells, NK cells, and plasma cells.[35] The binding of this agent to SLAMF-7 enhances the effects of the NK cells to cause antibody-dependent cellular cytotoxicity. This agent is indicated in combination with lenalidomide and dexamethasone for the treatment of MM in patients who have received 1 to 3 prior therapies based on higher PFS and ORR observed in clinical trials (see **Table 1**).[36] Elotuzumab is dosed at 10 mg/kg every week for the first 2 cycles, and then every 2 weeks subsequently. The risk of infusion reactions observed in clinical trials was 10%, therefore the manufacturer recommends that a histamine blocker and acetaminophen be given before therapy and provides a detailed steroid schedule. The infusion should be titrated up slowly to limit the potential for reactions following the parameters outlined in **Box 7**.

Liver enzyme levels should be monitored while patients are on this therapy; if increases are grade 3 or higher, therapy should be held until levels return to baseline values. An increased incidence of opportunistic infections was observed with this triple therapy in clinical trial, necessitating vigilant monitoring and prophylactic therapy as clinically indicated. Common ADEs are diarrhea, pyrexia, constipation, cough, peripheral neuropathy, nasopharyngitis, upper respiratory tract infections, decreased appetite, and pneumonia. In addition, there is a warning of a higher incidence of secondary primary malignancies. The clinical impact and follow-up have not been fully characterized, but this should remain a counseling point for patients. Similar to daratumumab, this therapy can affect the determination of complete response and possibly relapse from complete response in patients because of interference with assays used to monitor the M protein.

Box 7
Elotuzumab (Empliciti)

- Dose: 10 mg/kg intravenously every week for the first 2 cycles and every 2 weeks thereafter.
- Administration instructions: infusion titration is necessary for the first 2 doses.

Cycle	Time (min)	Rate (mL/min)
Cycle 1 Dose 1	0–30	0.5
	30–60	1
	60 or more	2
Cycle 1 Dose 2	0–30	1
	30 of more	2
Cycle 1 Dose 3 and 4	Any	2
Cycle 4 and greater	Any	May increase to 5

- Renal impairment: no clinical studies done in patients with severe renal impairment.
- Hepatic impairment: stop therapy on grade 3 or higher increase of liver enzyme levels. After return to baseline values, continuation of treatment may be considered.
- Monitoring:
  - CBC
  - LFT
  - Peripheral neuropathy
  - Infusion reactions
- Supportive care:
  - Premedications for infusion reactions as follows:
    - Dexamethasone
      - On the days elotuzumab is administered, give 28 mg of oral dexamethasone 3 to 24 hours before the infusion and 8 mg intravenous (IV) dexamethasone between 45 and 90 minutes before the infusion.
      - On days on which elotuzumab is not administered but a dose of dexamethasone is scheduled (days 8 and 22 of cycles 3 and onward), give 40 mg orally.
    - Diphenhydramine 25 to 50 mg oral or intravenously, or an equivalent H1 blocker
    - Ranitidine 50 mg intravenously or 150 mg orally, or an equivalent H2 blocker
    - Acetaminophen 650 to 1000 mg orally

IMMUNOTHERAPY

Immune checkpoints, including cytotoxic T lymphocyte–associated antigen 4 (CTLA-4) and programmed cell death receptor and its ligand (PD-1, PDL-1), are important targets for newly developed mAb therapy. Cancer cells have developed mechanisms of evading the innate ability of the immune system to identify malignant cells. CTLA-4 is active early in the stages of the immune response and primarily functions to reduce T-cell responses to self-antigens and prevent autoimmunity. The PD-1 protein is active in later stages and functions to stop ongoing immune activity.[37–39] Through this inhibition the body is able to detect the tumor cells that have evaded the immune system through antigen presentation impairment, secretion of immunosuppressive cells, and recruitment of inhibitory cells inducing T-cell nonresponsiveness. Patients with any underlying autoimmune condition are not candidates for therapy with immunotherapy because of the risk of an exacerbation of their condition.[40,41]

The first CTLA-4 checkpoint inhibitor, ipilimumab (Yervoy), was approved in 2011. The PD-1 inhibitors pembrolizumab (Keytruda) and nivolumab (Opdivo) were approved in 2014 and 2015.[42–44] All of these agents were initially approved for use in metastatic melanoma; however, ongoing clinical trials have resulted in breakthrough designations for metastatic NSCLC and renal cell carcinoma (RCC). There are also promising clinical trial data in hematologic malignancies and in combination with conventional cytotoxic chemotherapy regimens.

Ipilimumab was initially approved for unresectable or metastatic melanoma. In October of 2015 it received expanded approval for adjuvant melanoma treatment after resection in which lymph nodes were involved. Dosing for this expanded indication is reviewed in **Box 8**. These approvals are based on the positive impact ipilimumab had on median OS and recurrence-free survival in relapsed/refractory patients in the clinical trials (see **Table 1**).[45–47]

Pembrolizumab was the first PD-1 immune checkpoint inhibitor approved for relapsed/refractory metastatic melanoma in 2014. In 2015 its approval was expanded to first-line treatment of metastatic melanoma and metastatic NSCLC in patients whose tumors express PDL-1 after disease progression on or after platinum-containing chemotherapy. For both indications, therapy is given at 2 mg/kg every 3 weeks. Pembrolizumab proved to have more favorable PFS and ORR than conventional chemotherapy and prior therapy with ipilimumab. Further administration and monitoring specifics are detailed in **Box 9**.

Nivolumab was also initially approved for metastatic melanoma, but in less than a year its use has expanded to include metastatic NSCLC and advanced RCC, with various dosing specifics detailed in **Box 10**. In March of 2015, it also became the first agent indicated in combination with another immunotherapy agent with ipilimumab; the combination is indicated for the treatment of patients with unresectable or

---

Box 8
Ipilimumab (Yervoy)

- Doses:
  - Metastatic/unresectable melanoma: 3 mg/kg every 3 weeks for a maximum of 4 doses.
  - Adjuvant melanoma: 10 mg/kg every 3 weeks for 4 doses, then 10 mg/kg every 12 weeks for up to 3 years.

- Administration instructions: given intravenously over 90 minutes.

- Renal impairment: no clinical studies done in patients with severe renal impairment

- Hepatic impairment: hold therapy for aspartate transaminase (AST)/alanine transaminase (ALT) greater than 2.5 to less than or equal to 5 times the upper limit of normal (ULN) or bilirubin level greater than 1.5 to less than or equal to 3 times ULN. Permanently discontinue and administer corticosteroids for ALT or AST level greater than 5 times ULN, or total bilirubin level greater than 3 times ULN.

- Monitoring:
  - LFTs
  - Serum chemistries, including blood glucose, and adrenocorticotropic hormone
  - Thyroid-stimulating hormone
  - Signs of immune-related adverse events (irAEs) including hypophysitis, adrenal insufficiency, enterocolitis, rash, pruritus, motor or sensory neuropathy, and ocular toxicity

- Supportive care:
  - Systemic corticosteroids at 1 to 2 mg/kg prednisone equivalents for severe irAEs.
  - Loperamide and diphenoxylate and atropine as needed for mild diarrhea.
  - Topical steroids and antihistamines as needed for mild dermatitis.
  - Pregabalin, gabapentin, and/or pain medication as needed for peripheral neuropathy.
  - Appropriate hormone replacement as needed for immunotherapy-induced endocrinopathies.
  - Corticosteroid eye drops as needed for immunotherapy-induced uveitis.

Box 9
Pembrolizumab (Keytruda)

- Dose:
  - Metastatic/unresectable melanoma: 2 mg/kg every 3 weeks
  - Metastatic non–small cell lung cancer: 2 mg/kg once every 3 weeks following progression on or after platinum-containing chemotherapy.
- Administration instructions: given intravenously over 30 minutes.
- Renal impairment: no clinical studies done in patients with severe renal impairment.
- Hepatic impairment: hold therapy for AST/ALT greater than 3 to less than or equal to 5 times ULN or bilirubin level greater than 1.5 to less than 3 times ULN. Permanently discontinue and administer corticosteroids for ALT or AST level greater than 5 times ULN, or total bilirubin level greater than 3 times ULN.
- Monitoring: similar to ipilimumab, please refer to ipilimumab box.
- Supportive care: similar to ipilimumab, please refer to ipilimumab box.

---

metastatic melanoma. The mechanisms of action with respect to PD-1 blockade do not differ. Other than dosing schema and approved indications, there are no true differences that favor one agent more than another. However, the combination of nivolumab and ipilimumab inhibiting both PD-1 and CTLA-4 results in enhanced T-cell function that is greater than the effects of either antibody alone and results in improved antitumor responses in metastatic melanoma.

Immunotherapy is similar to conventional treatments in that shrinkage of baseline lesions, absence of new lesions, and durable stable disease can all be expected

---

Box 10
Nivolumab (Opdivo)

- Dose:
  - Relapsed/refractory metastatic/unresectable melanoma: 3 mg/kg every 2 weeks
  - First-line combination therapy metastatic/unresectable melanoma: 1 mg/kg every 3 weeks in combination with ipilimumab for 4 doses, followed by 3 mg/kg every 2 weeks as monotherapy
  - Metastatic non–small cell lung cancer: 3 mg/kg every 2 weeks following progression on or after platinum-containing chemotherapy
  - Advanced renal cell cancer: 3 mg/kg every 2 weeks following progression on antiangiogenic therapy
- Administration instructions: given intravenously over 60 minutes.
- Renal impairment: withhold treatment and consider systemic corticosteroids for creatinine level greater than 1.5 to 6 times ULN or greater than 1.5 times baseline. Permanently discontinue and administer systemic corticosteroids if creatinine level is greater than 6 times ULN.
- Hepatic impairment: hold therapy for AST/ALT greater than 3 to less than or equal to 5 times ULN or bilirubin level greater than 1.5 to less than 3 times ULN. Permanently discontinue and administer corticosteroids for ALT or AST level greater than 5 times ULN, or total bilirubin level greater than 3 times ULN.
- Monitoring: similar to ipilimumab, please refer to ipilimumab box.
- Supportive care: similar to ipilimumab, please refer to ipilimumab box.

---

with therapy. Immunotherapy differs in the time to effect and the possibility of pseudoprogression, the notion that the tumors and lesions may appear larger at first because of the higher number of immune cells infiltrating the tumor.[48] It takes time for the immune system to increase its scavenging ability, resulting in a slow and steady decline in tumor burden. This time-to-effect component should be considered in patients whose disease is rapidly evolving and requiring more immediate debulking.

Apart from the risk for infusion reactions, mAbs are fairly benign therapies that do not carry the typical side effects associated with cytotoxic chemotherapy. However, immunotherapy carries a risk for development of immune-related adverse events (irAEs). These side effects are unique to this therapy class and are related to autoimmune damage of various organ systems caused by the enhanced immune activity. Observations of these agents to date indicate that rates of grade 3 and 4 irAEs with PD-1 inhibition are lower compared with CTLA-4 inhibition. This finding is highlighted by ipilimumab carrying a black box warning for possibly fatal irAEs, whereas pembrolizumab and nivolumab only carry warnings and precautions for irAEs. The spectrum of irAEs patients can experience and their management are reviewed in **Table 2**.[42–44]

Patients who experience mild or moderate (grade 1 or 2) irAEs can be managed by holding immunotherapy and optimizing symptom management. If symptoms are more severe, therapy should be permanently held and high-dose corticosteroids at 1 to 2 mg/kg/d of a prednisone equivalent should be started and continued until the side effect downgrades in severity. The role of steroids in managing irAEs is to dampen the upregulated immune system. Steroids are not recommended to be given concurrently with immunotherapy at doses of greater than 10 mg of prednisone equivalents to avoid competing interests. Patients who remain on steroids at dosages equivalent to greater than or equal to 20 mg of prednisone daily for 1 month or longer should be given pneumocystis pneumonia prophylaxis.[49]

TYROSINE KINASE INHIBITORS

Similar to the advances in the use of mAbs as cancer treatments, there has been large growth in the availability and use of additional targeted therapies, such as small-molecule TKIs. There are more than 20 TKIs approved by the FDA, with 5 new approvals and 2 expanded indications in 2015.

Targeted therapy allows more direct selection of cancer cells while avoiding healthy, normal cells. Tyrosine kinases are a chief focus for drug development in oncology because of their involvement in growth factor signaling. Receptor tyrosine kinases are cell surface proteins that traverse the membrane and aid in transduction of extracellular signals to the cytoplasm. Nonreceptor tyrosine kinases transmit intracellular signals. Small-molecule TKIs correct the deregulation of the signaling cascade by opposing the tyrosine kinase phosphorylation and blocking the signaling pathway.

Imatinib (Gleevec) was the first approved TKI in 2001, targeting breakpoint cluster region of the gene "abl" (BCR-ABL) and revolutionizing treatment of chronic myelogenous leukemia. There has since been significant growth in available treatments with additional targeted TKIs. The new oral TKIs approved in 2015 are discussed here.

EPIDERMAL GROWTH FACTOR RECEPTOR INHIBITORS
Gefitinib

Gefitinib (Iressa) is a reversible inhibitor of wild-type and activating mutations of EGFR. It acts by preventing autophosphorylation of tyrosine residues associated with the receptor, thus inhibiting downstream signaling and blocking EGFR-dependent proliferation. Gefitinib originally received accelerated FDA approval in 2003 as first-line

Table 2
irAEs while on immunotherapy and their management

Side Effect	Grade 1 or 2 ADE	Grade 3 or 4 ADE
Enterocolitis	Withhold immunotherapy Provide symptomatic management Resume when ADE has resolved or is mild Consider steroids if symptoms persist >1 wk	Permanently discontinue immunotherapy Rule out bowel perforation Perform endoscopic evaluation *Give corticosteroids, 1–2 mg/kg/d prednisone equivalent* Continue steroids until symptoms improve, taper slowly for 1 mo
Hepatitis	Withhold immunotherapy when AST/ALT 2.5–5× ULN Resume therapy when labs <2.5× ULN	Permanently discontinue when AST/ALT >5× ULN *Give corticosteroids, 1–2 mg/kg/d prednisone equivalent* Continue steroids until labs improve, taper slowly for 1 mo
Dermatitis	Withhold immunotherapy Treat with topical steroids and/or antihistamines Resume when dermatitis resolves or improves	Permanently discontinue if SJS, TEN or other severe rash forms *Give corticosteroids, 1–2 mg/kg/d prednisone equivalent* Continue steroids until symptoms improve, taper slowly for 1 mo
Neurologic	Withhold immunotherapy Treat symptoms (pregabalin, gabapentin) Resume when symptoms resolve	Permanently discontinue if symptoms affect ADLs/life threatening Treat symptoms appropriately *Give corticosteroids, 1–2 mg/kg/d prednisone equivalent*
Endocrinopathy	Evaluate endocrine function Initiate appropriate hormone replacement therapy	Withhold immunotherapy in symptomatic patients *Give corticosteroids, 1–2 mg/kg/d prednisone equivalent* Initiate appropriate hormone replacement therapy Resume therapy when on ≤7.5 mg of prednisone equivalent daily
Uveitis	Typically resolves within 1 wk Consider corticosteroid eye drops	Consider systemic corticosteroids in severe cases
Pneumonitis	Perform imaging and evaluate lung function	Discontinue therapy Perform bronchoscopy, imaging, biopsies *Give corticosteroids, 1–2 mg/kg/d prednisone equivalent*

Abbreviations: labs, laboratory tests; SJS, steven johnson's syndrome; TEN, toxic epidermal necrosis.

monotherapy for locally advanced or metastatic NSCLC in patients who had failed both platinum-based and docetaxel chemotherapies. This approval was withdrawn when 2 postmarketing studies failed to show any significant survival benefit in either the overall study population or in patients with high levels of EGFR surface marker.[50]

In July 2015, the FDA approved gefitinib for first-line treatment of patients with metastatic NSCLC positive for EGFR exon 19 deletions or exon 21 (L858R) substitution mutations, becoming a treatment contender with erlotinib (Tarceva) and afatinib

(Gilotrif). Gefitinib's approval reinstatement was based on data from the Iressa Follow-Up Measure (IFUM) clinical trial and further supported by the Iressa Pan-Asia Study (IPASS) (**Table 3**).[51–53] From this analysis, it was concluded that EGFR mutations are the strongest predictive biomarker for PFS and tumor response to first-line gefitinib versus carboplatin/paclitaxel.

Similar to the anti-EGFR mAbs, patients should be monitored for common ADEs such as skin reactions (47%), nail conditions (5%), diarrhea (29%), vomiting (14%), stomatitis (7%), decreased appetite (17%), and conjunctivitis/blepharitis/dry eye (6%). Gefitinib should be held for up to 14 days if patients acutely develop or have worsening pulmonary symptoms, grade 2 or higher alanine transaminase (ALT)/aspartate transaminase (AST) increases, grade 3 or higher diarrhea, signs and symptoms of severe/worsening ocular disorders, or grade 3 or higher skin reactions. Treatment may be restarted on improvement to grade 1 or resolution of ADE. Gefitinib should be permanently discontinued should more serious complications, such as dermatologic toxicity, gastrointestinal perforation, ocular toxicity, and pulmonary toxicity occur. Signs and symptoms of ADEs should be monitored closely in CYP2D6 poor metabolizers and patients with hepatic impairment. In addition, strong CYP3A4 inhibitors may decrease gefitinib's metabolism. In concomitant use with strong CYP3A4 inducers, the dose of gefitinib should be increased to 500 mg daily. The standard recommended dose (**Box 11**) may be restarted 7 days after discontinuing the CYP3A4 inducer. The use of acid-suppressing drugs (proton pump inhibitors [PPIs], histamine H2–receptor antagonists, and antacids) may reduce plasma concentrations of gefitinib. If acid-suppression therapy is necessary, the use of antacids or H2 receptor blockers are preferred to PPIs. Administration of gefitinib should be separated from acid-suppression therapy to maximize absorption: gefitinib should be administered 6 hours before or after H2 receptor antagonist or antacid, or 12 hours before or after a PPI.

Despite the discovery of gefitinib's role in this specific patient population, its effects are short lived because most patients develop resistance to EGFR-specific TKIs and relapse.[60,61] Studies are currently underway investigating how to better manage and possibly prevent this development of resistance.

Osimertinib

Osimertinib (Tagrisso) was designed to target the EGFR T790M mutation present in approximately 50% to 60% of cases of acquired TKI resistance in NSCLC.[62,63] This third-generation EGFR TKI was approved in November 2015 for metastatic EGFR T790M mutation-positive NSCLC with disease progression despite EGFR TKI therapy (see **Table 3** for clinical trial data). T790M EGFR mutation must be confirmed.[54] Continued approval for this indication may be contingent on further confirmatory studies. **Box 12** provides dosing details.

The most common ADEs are diarrhea (42%), rash (41%), dry skin (31%), and nail toxicity (25%). Nail toxicity may present as redness, tenderness, pain, inflammation, brittleness, separation from nail bed, and desquamation of nails. Osimertinib should be held up to 4 weeks in patients with asymptomatic, and absolute decrease in left ventricular ejection fraction (LVEF) of 10% from baseline and less than 50%. It may be restarted on improvement to baseline. Any grade 3 or higher ADE warrants holding of treatment for up to 3 weeks, resuming with improvement to grade 0 to 2 at 80 mg or 40 mg daily. Osimertinib should be held in patients experiencing QTc prolongation (QTc interval >500 milliseconds on 2 separate electrocardiograms). Once the QTc interval is less than 481 milliseconds or there is recovery to baseline, osimertinib may be restarted at a dose of 40 mg. Therapy should be permanently stopped for any of the following: interstitial lung disease/pneumonitis, QTc interval prolongation with

Table 3
Summary of clinical trials of TKIs

Drug	Study Design	Population	Results
Gefitinib (Iressa)	IFUM[52] Prospective, open-label, multicenter, single-arm study, (n = 107) Gefitinib 250 mg/d	Untreated EGFR mutation-positive, locally advanced or metastatic NSCLC	• ORR ○ Investigator Assessment (IA) 69.8% (95% CI: 60.5%–77.7%) ○ Blind Independent Central Review (BICR) 50.0% (95% CI: 40.6%–59.4%) • Median DOR ○ IA 6.0 mo (95% CI: 5.6–11.1) ○ BICR 8.3 mo (95% CI: 7.6–11.3)
	IPASS[53] Phase 3, open-label study, RCT (n = 1217) Gefitinib 250 mg/d (G) vs carboplatin (AUC 5–6) + paclitaxel (200 mg/m²) (CP)	Untreated stage IIIB–IV pulmonary adenocarcinoma Light-never smokers	• ORR ○ G 67% (95% CI: 56–77) vs CP 41% (95% CI: 31–51) • Median PFS ○ G 10.9 mo vs CP 7.4 mo ○ HR of 0.54 (95% CI: 0.38, 0.79) • Median DOR ○ G 9.6 mo vs CP 5.5 mo
Osimertinib (Tagrisso)	• Two multicenter, single-arm, open-label clinical trials (n = 411)[54] ○ Study 1: n = 201 ○ Study 2: n = 210	Advanced EGFR T790M mutation-positive NSCLC with disease progression after treatment with an EGFR TKI	• ORR ○ Overall: 59% ○ Study 1: 57% ○ Study 2: 61% • Ongoing response ○ 96% of patients with a confirmed objective response had an ongoing response ranging from 1.1–5.6 mo ○ Median duration follow-up ○ Study 1: 4.2 mo ○ Study 2: 4.0 mo
	Preliminary data from the AURA phase I trial first-line cohort and 2 AURA phase II studies, (n = 60)[70]	First-line in EGFRm-positive advanced NSCLC and previously treated patients with EGFRm T790M mutation-positive NSCLC	• PFS ○ 72% (95% CI: 58%–82%) at 12 mo • ORR ○ 75% (95% CI: 62%–85%) • DOR ○ 18 mo and ongoing

(continued on next page)

Table 3
(continued)

Drug	Study Design	Population	Results
Cobimetinib (Cotellic)	coBRIM study phase III multicenter, RCT (n = 495)[55] Vemurafenib 960 mg orally BID days 1–28 + cobimetinib 60 mg (VC) or matching placebo orally (VP) once daily days 1–21 of an every 28-d cycle	Untreated BRAF V600 mutation-positive, unresectable, or metastatic melanoma	• Median PFS ○ VC 12.3 mo (95% CI: 9.5–13.4) ○ VP 7.2 mo (95% CI: 5.6–7.5) ○ HR 0.56 (95% CI: 0.45–0.70) • Median OS ○ VC NE (95% CI: 20.7–NE) ○ VP 17.0 mo (95% CI: 15.0–NE) ○ HR 0.63 (95% CI: 0.47–0.85) • ORR ○ VC 70% (95% CI: 64%–75%) ○ VP 50% (95% CI: 44%–56%) • Median DOR ○ VC 13.0 mo (95% CI: 11.1–16.6) ○ VP 9.2 mo (95% CI: 7.5–12.8)

Abbreviations: BID, twice a day; DCR, disease control rate (defined by CR plus PR plus stable disease for 6 weeks); DOR, duration of response; NE, not estimable; ORR, overall response rate.

signs/symptoms of life-threatening arrhythmia, symptomatic congestive heart failure, or grade 3 or higher ADE with no improvement within 3 weeks. Effective contraception should be used during treatment. It is recommended that women should continue use for 6 weeks after their final dose and for men to use effective birth control for 4 months after their final dose.

Box 11
Gefitinib (Iressa)

• Dose: 250 mg orally once daily until disease progression or unacceptable toxicity

• Administration instructions: with or without food; may be dissolved in 124 to 240 mL (4 to 8 ounces) of water (let dissolve for ~15 minutes; drink liquid immediately)

• Renal impairment: no clinical studies done in patients with severe renal impairment

• Hepatic impairment: no dose adjustments recommended; monitor ADEs in patients with moderate to severe impairment

• Monitoring:
  ○ EGFR mutation status
  ○ LFTs
  ○ Renal function
  ○ Electrolytes

• Supportive care: ADE management as needed

Box 12
Osimertinib (Tagrisso)

- Dose: 80 mg orally daily

- Administration instructions: with or without food; may be dissolved in ~ 50 mL of noncarbonated water; stir until completely dispersed and administer immediately

- Renal impairment: no dose adjustment recommended in mild (CrCl, 60–89 mL/min) or moderate (CrCl, 30–59 mL/min) renal impairment; no recommended dose for severe renal impairment (CrCl <30 mL/min) or end-stage renal disease

- Hepatic impairment: no dose adjustment is recommended in mild hepatic impairment; no recommended dose for moderate or severe hepatic impairment

- Monitoring:
  - EGFR mutation status
  - Left ventricular ejection fraction (LVEF) (echo/muga)
  - Electrocardiograms (ECGs) and electrolytes
  - CBC

Abbreviation: ECHO/MUGA, echocardiogram/multigated acquisition scan.

Concurrent administration of strong CYP3A4 inducers and inhibitors should be avoided. If the use of CYP3A4 inhibitors is unavoidable, patients should be monitored closely for signs of toxicity. Osimertinib may increase or decrease plasma concentrations of substrates of CYP3A, breast cancer resistance protein (BCRP), or CYP1A2.

MITOGEN/EXTRACELLULAR SIGNAL REGULATED KINASE INHIBITORS
Cobimetinib

BRAF inhibitors have made a significant impact on the treatment of melanoma. However, 80% of tumors develop BRAF inhibitor resistance via reactivation of mitogen-activated protein kinase (MAPK) signaling. Mitogen/extracellular signal regulated kinase (MEK) inhibitors can target MAPK-dependent tumors and thus have become an integral part of combination therapy in BRAF-mutated melanoma.[64]

Cobimetinib (Cotellic) is a reversible MAPK, MEK1, and MEK2 inhibitor. It gained FDA approval in November 2015 as combination treatment with vemurafenib (Zelboraf) in unresectable or metastatic melanoma with BRAF V600E or V600K mutation (see **Table 3**). Cobimetinib should not be used in patients with wild-type BRAF melanoma.[58] **Box 13** shows dosing details.

Common ADEs with this medication regimen include diarrhea (60%), photosensitivity reaction (46%), nausea (41%), pyrexia (28%), and vomiting (24%). The most common (≥5%) grade 3 to 4 laboratory abnormalities were increased gamma-glutamyl transferase level, increased creatine phosphokinase (CPK) level, hypophosphatemia, increased ALT level, lymphopenia, increased AST level, increased alkaline phosphatase level, and hyponatremia. Patients should also be monitored for severe dermatologic reactions, hepatotoxicity, and rhabdomyolysis, which require dose interruption and subsequent dose reduction. There is a risk of developing new cutaneous and noncutaneous primary malignancies during therapy and up to 6 months after discontinuation. Serious hemorrhagic effects, retinal vein occlusion, and symptomatic LVEF decrease from baseline warrant permanent discontinuation of cobimetinib. The incidence of cardiomyopathy is higher in patients on combination cobimetinib and vemurafenib compared with single-agent vemurafenib. At present no recommendations exist for its safety in patients with decreased LVEF at baseline. LVEF should be monitored before treatment, at 1 month, then every 3 months during treatment.

Box 13
Cobimetinib (Cotellic)

- Dose: 60 mg orally once daily for the first 21 days of each 28-day cycle until disease progression or unacceptable toxicity.

- Administration instructions: with or without food.

- Renal impairment: no dose adjustment is recommended for mild to moderate renal impairment (CrCl, 30–89 mL/min); there is no recommended dose for patients with severe renal impairment.

- Hepatic impairment: no dose adjustment is recommended in mild hepatic impairment (total bilirubin level ≤ULN and AST level >ULN or total bilirubin >ULN but ≤1.5 times ULN and any AST level). Dose reductions are recommended for hepatotoxicity.

- Monitoring:
  - BRAF mutation status
  - LFTs
  - LVEF
  - ECGs and electrolytes
  - CBC

- Supportive care: antiemetics as needed

Necessary dose reductions may be done in a stepwise fashion: first dose reduction to 40 mg, second dose reduction to 20 mg, and third or subsequent reductions resulting in discontinuation of cobimetinib.

Cobimetinib is a CYP3A4 substrate. Concomitant use of strong or moderate CYP3A inducers or inhibitors should be avoided. If it is medically necessary to use a moderate CYP3A4 inhibitor in the short term (≤14 days) for patients who are taking cobimetinib 60 mg, the cobimetinib dose should be reduced to 20 mg. In patients who are already taking a reduced dose of cobimetinib, an alternative to the strong or moderate CYP3A4 inhibitor should be sought. After therapy with a moderate CYP3A inhibitor is complete, the previous 60-mg dose of cobimetinib may be restarted.

Miscellaneous Targeted Therapy

In addition to mAbs and TKIs, several medications with other mechanisms were approved in 2015. These various oncology agents with novel mechanisms that gained approval in 2015 are discussed here. In addition, a discussion of newly approved miscellaneous agents that revitalize established mechanisms of action, including lenvatinib, ixazomib, trifluridine/tipiracil, and trabectedin, is provided in the Supplemental Material.

CYCLIN-DEPENDENT KINASE INHIBITOR
Palbociclib

Cyclin-dependent kinases promote progression through the cell cycle by phosphorylating downstream proteins. Palbociclib (Ibrance) inhibits CDK4 and CDK6, halting cell replication. It has shown synergy with antiestrogen therapies.[65–70] Palbociclib received FDA approval in February 2015 for the treatment of estrogen receptor (ER)–positive, human EGF receptor 2 (HER2)–negative breast cancer in combination with letrozole in postmenopausal women as initial hormonal therapy for advanced disease.[65] Palbociclib has also been studied in combination with fulvestrant in previously treated ER-positive breast cancer (**Table 4**).[66]

The use of palbociclib is limited by high rates of neutropenia, reported in more than 75% of patients in clinical trials. Grade 3 or greater neutropenia occurred in more than

Table 4
Summary of clinical trials of miscellaneous targeted agents in oncology

Drug	Study Design	Population	Results
Palbociclib (Ibrance)	PALOMA 1: phase 2, open-label, RCT comparing PL with L, n = 165	Initial therapy for advanced ER + breast cancer in postmenopausal women	• Median PFS: 20.2 vs 10.2 mo favoring PL ○ HR: 0.488 (95% CI 0.319–0.748; P = .0004) • ORR: 43% vs 33% favoring PL ○ P = .13 • Median DOR: 20.3 vs 11.1 mo favoring PL • Median OS: 37.5 vs 33.3 mo favoring PL ○ HR: 0.813 (95% CI 0.492–1.345; P = .42)
	PALOMA 3: phase 3, double-blind RCT comparing P + F with placebo + F, n = 521	Advanced hormone receptor + breast cancer R/R to endocrine therapy	• Median PFS: 9.2 vs 3.8 mo favoring P + F ○ HR: 0.42 (95% CI 0.32–0.56; P<.001) • ORR: 10.4% vs 6.3% favoring P + F ○ P = .16 • CBR: 34.0% vs 19.0% favoring P + F ○ P<.001 • OS: pending
Panobinostat (Farydak)	PANORAMA2[59]: phase 2 open-label trial of panobinostat in combination with bortezomib and dexamethasone, n = 55	Relapsed and bortezomib-refractory MM with ≥2 lines prior therapy including an immunomodulatory drug	• ORR: 34.5% • Median DOR: 6.0 mo • Median PFS: 5.4 mo • Median OS: not reached
	PANORAMA1[57]: phase 3, double-blind RCT comparing panobinostat or PBD or BD), n = 768	RR MM with 1–3 prior treatments	• Median PFS: 11.99 vs 8.08 mo favoring PBD ○ HR: 0.63 (95% CI 0.52–0.76; P<.0001) • Median OS: 33.64 vs 30.39 mo favoring PBD (interim analysis) ○ HR 0.87 (95% CI 0.69–1.10; P = .26) • ORR: 60.7% vs 54.6% favoring PBD • Median DOR: 13.14 vs 10.87 mo favoring PBD
Sonidegib (Odomzo)	BOLT: phase 2, double-blind RCT comparing 2 doses of sonidegib (200 mg vs 800 mg), n = 230	Locally advanced or metastatic BCC not treatable with radiation or surgery	• ORR: 36% vs 34% • Median DOR: not calculated ○ Responses lasting ≥6 mo: 39% vs 38% • DCR: 84% vs 96%

Abbreviations: BCC, basal cell carcinoma; CBR, clinical benefit rate (CR plus PR plus prolonged stable disease); DCR, disease control rate (CR plus PR plus stable disease); F, fulvestrant; L, letrozole; PBD, placebo in combination with bortezomib and dexamethasone; P + F, palbociclib + fulvestrant; PFS, progression-free survival; PL, palbociclib plus letrozole; RCT, randomized control trial.

half of patients, with febrile neutropenia occurring rarely. Additional common hematologic toxicities included anemia and thrombocytopenia[66,67] Nonhematologic toxicities occurring in more than 20% of patients were fatigue, nausea, diarrhea, stomatitis, arthralgia, alopecia, hot flushes, and headache.[65–67]

Palbociclib is given once daily on days 1 to 21 of a 28-day cycle. Detailed dosing and administration information is contained in **Box 14**. Palbociclib undergoes extensive hepatic metabolism via CYP3A4. Concomitant use of strong CYP3A4 inhibitors and strong and moderate CYP3A4 inducers should be avoided. If strong inhibitors cannot be avoided, the dose of palbociclib should be reduced. In addition, palbociclib inhibits CYP3A4, therefore substrates of this enzyme with a narrow therapeutic index should be avoided during treatment. Palbociclib has the potential to cause embryofetal toxicity. Women of childbearing potential should use effective contraception during treatment and for 2 weeks following discontinuation.[65]

HISTONE DEACETYLASE INHIBITORS
Panobinostat

Histone deacetylase (HDAC) enzymes have activity in cell cycle regulation. HDAC inhibitors cause cell cycle arrest and apoptosis because of accumulation of acetylated histones and proteins. There are currently 4 HDAC inhibitors approved by the FDA: vorinostat (Zolinza, 2006), romidepsin (Istodax, 2009), belinostat (Beleodaq, 2014), and panobinostat (Farydak, 2015). Vorinostat, romidepsin, and belinostat are approved for T-cell lymphomas. Panobinostat is indicated for the treatment of MM in patients who have received at least 2 prior regimens that contained bortezomib and an immunomodulatory agent.[56] Accelerated approval was granted in February 2015 based on PFS in combination with bortezomib and dexamethasone (see **Table 4**).[57] Confirmatory trials are ongoing.

Panobinostat carries black box warnings for diarrhea and cardiac toxicities. Diarrhea was reported in as many as 68% of patients in clinical trials, with grade 3 to 4 diarrhea occurring in 25% of patients.[57] This adverse event should be aggressively managed with antidiarrheal medications such as loperamide. Arrhythmias and cardiac ischemic events were reported at higher rates in patients receiving panobinostat than in comparator arms.[56] Patients should be carefully selected and monitored for cardiac toxicities and electrolyte abnormalities during treatment. Additional severe ADEs reported include hemorrhage, myelosuppression, infections, and hepatotoxicity. The most common ADEs in patients receiving treatment with panobinostat, bortezomib, and dexamethasone were diarrhea, fatigue, nausea, decreased appetite, pyrexia, vomiting, and cough.[56,57,59] Peripheral neuropathy occurred at similar rates in panobinostat and placebo arms and was likely attributable to bortezomib.[57]

Box 14
Palbociclib (Ibrance)

- Dose: 125 mg orally once daily days 1 to 21 of a 28-day cycle
- Renal impairment: no adjustment
- Hepatic impairment: no adjustment
- Administration instructions: with food
- Monitoring: CBC
- Supportive care: consider antiemetic

Panobinostat is administered in a dosage of 20 mg orally 3 times weekly during weeks 1 and 2 of a 3-week cycle (**Box 15**). Panobinostat is a CYP3A substrate and CYP2D6 inducer. Use of strong CYP3A inducers and inhibitors should be avoided during panobinostat treatment. If coadministration of panobinostat and strong CYP3A inhibitors is medically necessary, panobinostat should be administered at a dose of 10 mg. Avoid coadministration with CYP2D6 substrates with narrow therapeutic indexes.[56]

HEDGEHOG PATHWAY INHIBITOR
Sonidegib

Mutations in the hedgehog pathway lead to uncontrolled basal cell proliferation and are present in most basal cell carcinomas (BCCs). These mutations typically occur in the transmembrane proteins Patched (PTCH1) or Smoothened (SMO), leading to activated transcription factors and cellular proliferation.[71,72] Vismodegib (Erivedge) was the first hedgehog pathway inhibitor available in the United States when approved in 2012. The FDA approval of sonidegib (Odomzo) in July 2015 provided a second agent in this class. Sonidegib and vismodegib inhibit SMO, preventing activation of this pathway.[71,72] Both agents are indicated to treat locally advanced BCC that recurred after radiation or surgery or in patients who are not candidates for radiation or surgery.[71,73]

Musculoskeletal reactions, including muscle spasms, increased creatine kinase (CK) level, myalgia, and arthralgia, were reported in more than 10% of patients taking sonidegib. Rhabdomyolysis has also been reported. CK levels should be monitored at baseline and periodically, especially in patients reporting muscle-related adverse reactions. Gastrointestinal side effects are also common, with nausea and diarrhea reported in more than 20% of patients. Other common adverse reactions included alopecia, dysgeusia, fatigue, weight loss, and decreased appetite. Common laboratory abnormalities were increased creatinine level, increased lipase level, hyperglycemia, anemia, and lymphopenia.[72]

Sonidegib can cause fetal death or severe birth defects if given to pregnant women. Women should avoid pregnancy during treatment and for 20 months after discontinuing sonidegib, and men should use condoms during treatment and for 8 months after

---

Box 15
Panobinostat (Farydak)

- Dose: 20 mg orally 3 times weekly during weeks 1 and 2 of a 3-week cycle (days 1, 3, 5, 8, 10, 12, and every 21 days)

- Renal impairment: no adjustment

- Hepatic impairment: reduce initial dose (15 mg in mild impairment, 10 mg in moderate impairment)

- Administration instructions: with or without food

- Monitoring:
  - CBC
  - LFTs
  - Electrolytes
  - ECG

- Supportive care:
  - Consider antiemetic
  - Acyclovir (because of coadministration with bortezomib)

Box 16
Sonidegib (Odomzo)

- Dose: 200 mg orally daily
- Renal impairment: no adjustment
- Hepatic impairment: no adjustment
- Administration instructions: take on an empty stomach
- Monitoring:
  - CK
  - Creatinine
  - Pregnancy test
- Supportive care: consider antiemetic and antidiarrheal

---

discontinuation. Patients should not donate blood while taking sonidegib or for 20 months after discontinuation.[71]

Sonidegib is administered at a daily dose of 200 mg (**Box 16**). Absorption of sonidegib is affected by high-fat meals and acid-suppression therapy. It should be taken on an empty stomach and medications such as PPIs and H2 blockers should be avoided. Metabolism occurs through the CYP3A4 pathway; coadministration with strong and moderate CYP3A4 inhibitors and inducers should be avoided.[71]

SUMMARY

Extensive progress has been made in targeted therapy in the last 10 years and its growth and progression have continued significantly in the year 2015. Although oncology health care providers continue to gain tools in their anticancer armamentarium, it is important to remember that many of these new agents have been granted accelerated approval based on surrogate end points. Continued approval of these agents depends on verification of clinical outcomes. In addition, providers must remain vigilant in optimizing supportive care therapies because of the unique side effect profiles of immunotherapy and shifting of oncology care to the outpatient setting with oral oncolytic therapies.

SUPPLEMENTARY DATA

Supplementary data related to this article can be found at http://dx.doi.org/10.1016/j.cpha.2016.03.012.

REFERENCES

1. Scott AM, Allison JP, Wolchok JD. Monoclonal antibodies in cancer therapy. Cancer Immun 2012;12:14.
2. Food and Drug Administration. Hematology/oncology (cancer) approvals & safety notifications. Available at: Http://www.fda.gov/Drugs/InformationOnDrugs/ApprovedDrugs. Accessed January 28, 2016.
3. Scott AM, Wolchok JD, Old LJ. Antibody therapy of cancer. Nat Rev Cancer 2012; 12(4):278–87.
4. Liu JK. The history of monoclonal antibody development - Progress, remaining challenges and future innovations. Ann Med Surg (Lond) 2014;3(4):113–6.
5. Chames P, Van Regenmortel M, Weiss E, et al. Therapeutic antibodies: successes, limitations and hopes for the future. Br J Pharmacol 2009;157(2):220–33.

6. Geskin LJ. Monoclonal antibodies. Dermatol Clin 2015;33(4):777–86.
7. Imai K, Takaoka A. Comparing antibody and small-molecule therapies for cancer. Nat Rev Cancer 2006;6(9):714–27.
8. American Medical Association. Monoclonal antibodies. Web. 30 Jan. 2016. Available at: http://www.ama-assn.org/ama/pub/physician-resources/medical-science/united-states-adopted-names-council/naming-guidelines/naming-biologics/monoclonal-antibodies.page?.
9. Newland AM, Li JX, Wasco LE, et al. Brentuximab vedotin: a CD30-directed anti-body-cytotoxic drug conjugate. Pharmacotherapy 2013;33(1):93–104.
10. Adcetris [package insert]. Bothell, WA: Seattle Genetics; 2015.
11. National Comprehensive Cancer Network (NCCN). NCCN clinical practice guidelines in antiemesis. Version 2. Washington, PA: National Comprehensive Cancer Network; 2015.
12. Carson KR, Newsome SD, Kim EJ, et al. Progressive multifocal leukoencephalopathy associated with brentuximab vedotin therapy: a report of 5 cases from the Southern Network on Adverse Reactions (SONAR) project. Cancer 2014; 120(16):2464–71.
13. Food and Drug Administration. U.S. Food and Drug Administration drug development and drug interactions: table of substrates, Inhibitors and Inducers. 27 Oct. 2014. Web. Available at: http://www.fda.gov/Drugs/DevelopmentApproval Process/DevelopmentResources/DrugInteractionsLabeling/ucm093664.htm.
14. Darzalex [package insert]. Horsham, PA: Janssen Biotech; 2015.
15. Lokhorst HM, Plesner T, Laubach JP, et al. Targeting CD38 with daratumumab monotherapy in multiple myeloma. N Engl J Med 2015;373(13):1207–19.
16. Avastin [package insert]. South San Francisco, CA: Genentech; 2015.
17. Cyramza [package insert]. Indianapolis, IN: Eli Lily; 2015.
18. Fuchs CS, Tomasek J, Yong CJ, et al. Ramucirumab monotherapy for previously treated advanced gastric or gastro-oesophageal junction adenocarcinoma (RE-GARD): an international, randomised, multicentre, placebo-controlled, phase 3 trial. Lancet 2014;383(9911):31–9.
19. Tabernero J, Yoshino T, Cohn AL, et al. Ramucirumab versus placebo in combination with second-line FOLFIRI in patients with metastatic colorectal carcinoma that progressed during or after first-line therapy with bevacizumab, oxaliplatin, and a fluoropyrimidine (RAISE): a randomised, double-blind, multicentre, phase 3 study. Lancet Oncol 2015;16(5):499–508.
20. Garon EB, Ciuleanu TE, Arrieta O, et al. Ramucirumab plus docetaxel versus placebo plus docetaxel for second-line treatment of stage IV non-small-cell lung cancer after disease progression on platinum-based therapy (REVEL): a multi-centre, double-blind, randomised phase 3 trial. Lancet 2014;384(9944):665–73.
21. Wilke H, Muro K, Van Cutsem E, et al. Ramucirumab plus paclitaxel versus placebo plus paclitaxel in patients with previously treated advanced gastric or gastro-oesophageal junction adenocarcinoma (RAINBOW): a double-blind, randomised phase 3 trial. Lancet Oncol 2014;15(11):1224–35.
22. Launay-Vacher V, Deray G. Hypertension and proteinuria: a class-effect of antiangiogenic therapies. Anticancer Drugs 2009;20(1):81–2.
23. Ciardiello F, Tortora G. EGFR antagonists in cancer treatment. N Engl J Med 2008; 358(11):1160–74.
24. Erbitux [package insert]. Indianapolis, IN: Eli Lilly; 2015.
25. Portrazza [package insert]. Indianapolis, IN: Eli Lilly; 2015.
26. Thatcher N, Hirsch FR, Luft AV, et al. Necitumumab plus gemcitabine and cisplatin versus gemcitabine and cisplatin alone as first-line therapy in patients

with stage IV squamous non-small-cell lung cancer (SQUIRE): an open-label, randomised, controlled phase 3 trial. Lancet Oncol 2015;16(7):763–74.

27. Paz-Ares L, Mezger J, Ciuleanu TE, et al. Necitumumab plus pemetrexed and cisplatin as first-line therapy in patients with stage IV non-squamous non-small-cell lung cancer (INSPIRE): an open-label, randomised, controlled phase 3 study. Lancet Oncol 2015;16(3):328–37.

28. Maliakal P, Ledford A. Electrolyte and protein imbalance following anti-EGFR therapy in cancer patients: A comparative study. Exp Ther Med 2010;1(2):307–11.

29. Chanprapaph K, Vachiramon V, Rattanakaemakorn P. Epidermal growth factor receptor inhibitors: a review of cutaneous adverse events and management. Dermatol Res Pract 2014;2014:734249.

30. Melosky B, Burkes R, Rayson D, et al. Management of skin rash during EGFR-targeted monoclonal antibody treatment for gastrointestinal malignancies: Canadian recommendations. Curr Oncol 2009;16(1):16–26.

31. Lacouture ME, Anadkat MJ, Bensadoun RJ, et al. Clinical practice guidelines for the prevention and treatment of EGFR inhibitor-associated dermatologic toxicities. Support Care Cancer 2011;19(8):1079–95.

32. Bianchini D, Jayanth A, Chua YJ, et al. Epidermal growth factor receptor inhibitor-related skin toxicity: mechanisms, treatment, and its potential role as a predictive marker. Clin Colorectal Cancer 2008;7(1):33–43.

33. Blincyto [package insert]. Thousand Oaks, CA: Amgen; 2015.

34. Topp MS, Gökbuget N, Stein AS, et al. Safety and activity of blinatumomab for adult patients with relapsed or refractory B-precursor acute lymphoblastic leukaemia: a multicentre, single-arm, phase 2 study. Lancet Oncol 2015;16(1): 57–66.

35. Empliciti [package insert]. Princeton, NJ: Bristol-Myers Squibb; 2015.

36. Lonial S, Dimopoulos M, Palumbo A, et al. Elotuzumab therapy for relapsed or refractory multiple myeloma. N Engl J Med 2015;373(7):621–31.

37. Lu J, Lee-Gabel L, Nadeau MC, et al. Clinical evaluation of compounds targeting PD-1/PD-L1 pathway for cancer immunotherapy. J Oncol Pharm Pract 2015; 21(6):451–67.

38. Davies M. New modalities of cancer treatment for NSCLC: focus on immunotherapy. Cancer Manag Res 2014;6:63–75.

39. Drake CG, Lipson EJ, Brahmer JR. Breathing new life into immunotherapy: review of melanoma, lung and kidney cancer. Nat Rev Clin Oncol 2014;11(1):24–37.

40. Yoon SH. Immunotherapy for non-small cell lung cancer. Tuberc Respir Dis (Seoul) 2014;77(3):111–5.

41. Langer CJ. Emerging immunotherapies in the treatment of non-small cell lung cancer (NSCLC): the role of immune checkpoint inhibitors. Am J Clin Oncol 2015;38(4):422–30.

42. Opdivo [package insert]. Princeton, NJ: Bristol-Myers Squibb; 2015.

43. Keytruda [package insert]. Whitehouse Station, NJ: Merck & Co; 2015.

44. Yervoy [package insert]. Princeton, NJ: Bristol-Myers Squibb; 2015.

45. Robert C, Thomas L, Bondarenko I, et al. Ipilimumab plus dacarbazine for previously untreated metastatic melanoma. N Engl J Med 2011;364(26):2517–26.

46. Hodi FS, O'Day SJ, McDermott DF, et al. Improved survival with ipilimumab in patients with metastatic melanoma. N Engl J Med 2010;363(8):711–23.

47. Robert C, Ribas A, Wolchok JD, et al. Anti-programmed-death-receptor-1 treatment with pembrolizumab in ipilimumab-refractory advanced melanoma: a randomised dose-comparison cohort of a phase 1 trial. Lancet 2014;384(9948): 1109–17.

48. Ott PA, Hodi FS, Robert C. CTLA-4 and PD-1/PD-L1 blockade: new immunother-apeutic modalities with durable clinical benefit in melanoma patients. Clin Cancer Res 2013;19(19):5300–9.

49. Tarhini A. Immune-mediated adverse events associated with ipilimumab CTLA-4 blockade therapy: the underlying mechanisms and clinical management. Scien-tifica (Cairo) 2013;2013:857519.

50. US Food and Drug Administration, Center for Drug Evaluation and Research. Infor-mation for Healthcare Professionals: Gefitinib (marketed as Iressa), FDA ALERT [6/2005]. Available at: http://www.fda.gov/Drugs/DrugSafety/PostmarketDrugSafety InformationforPatientsandProviders/DrugSafetyInformationforHeathcareProfessionals/ucm085197.htm. Accessed January 31, 2016.

51. Iressa [package insert]. Wilmington, DE: AstraZeneca Pharmaceuticals LP; 2015.

52. Douillard JY, Ostoros G, Cobo M, et al. First-line gefitinib in Caucasian EGFR mutation-positive NSCLC patients: a phase-IV, open-label, single-arm study. Br J Cancer 2014;110:55–62.

53. Fukuoka M, Wu YL, Thongprasert S, et al. Biomarker analyses and final overall survival results from a phase III, randomized, open-label, first-line study of gefiti-nib versus carboplatin/paclitaxel in clinically selected patients with advanced non-small-cell lung cancer in Asia (IPASS). J Clin Oncol 2011;29(21):2866–74.

54. Tagrisso [package insert]. Wilmington, DE: AstraZeneca Pharmaceuticals LP; 2015.

55. Larkin JMG, Yan Y, McArthur GA, et al. Update of progression-free survival (PFS) and correlative biomarker analysis from coBRIM: Phase III study of cobimetinib (cobi) plus vemurafenib (vem) in advanced BRAF-mutated melanoma. J Clin On-col 2015;33(Suppl) [Abstract 9006].

56. Farydak (panobinostat) [package insert]. East Hanover, NJ: Novartis Pharmaceu-ticals Corporation; 2015.

57. San-Miguel JF, Hungria VT, Yoon SS, et al. Panobinostat plus bortezomib and dexamethasone versus placebo plus bortezomib and dexamethasone in patients with relapsed or relapsed and refractory multiple myeloma: a multicentre, rando-mised, double-blind phase 3 trial. Lancet Oncol 2014;15:1195–206.

58. Cotellic [package insert]. South San Francisco, CA: Genetech USA; 2015.

59. Richardson PG, Schlossman RL, Alsina M, et al. PANORAMA 2: panobinostat in combination with bortezomib and dexamethasone in patients with relapsed and bortezomib-refractory myeloma. Blood 2013;122(14):2331–7.

60. Ogino A, Kitao H, Hirano S, et al. Emergence of epidermal growth factor receptor T790M mutation during chronic exposure to gefitinib in a non–small cell lung can-cer cell line. Cancer Res 2011;67:7807.

61. Ware KE, Hinz TK, Kleczko E, et al. A mechanism of resistance to gefitinib medi-ated by cellular reprogramming and the acquisition of an FGF2-FGFR1 autocrine growth loop. Oncogenesis 2013;2:e39.

62. Kobayashi S, Boggon TJ, Dayaram T, et al. EGFR mutation and resistance of non-small-cell lung cancer to gefitinib. N Engl J Med 2005;352(8):786–92.

63. Pao W, Miller VA, Politi KA, et al. Acquired resistance of lung adenocarcinomas to gefitinib or erlotinib is associated with a second mutation in the EGFR kinase domain. PLoS Med 2005;2(3):e73.

64. Tran KA, Cheng MY, Mitra A, et al. MEK inhibitors and their potential in the treat-ment of advanced melanoma: the advantages of combination therapy. Drug Des Devel Ther 2016;10:43–52.

65. Ibrance (palbociclib) [package insert]. New York, NY: Pfizer; 2015.

66. Turner NC, Ro J, Andre F, et al. Palbociclib in hormone-receptor-positive advanced breast cancer. N Engl J Med 2015;373:209–19.
67. Finn RS, Crown JP, Lang I, et al. The cyclin-dependent kinase 4/6 inhibitor palbociclib in combination with letrozole versus letrozole alone as first-line treatment of oestrogen receptor-positive, HER2-negative, advanced breast cancer (PALOMA-1/TRIO-18): a randomised phase 2 study. Lancet Oncol 2015;16:25–35.
68. Yang JC, Ahn M, Ramalingam SS, et al. AZD9291 in pre-treated T790M positive advanced NSCLC: AURA study phase II extension cohort [abstract]. Presented at the 16th World Conference on Lung Cancer. Denver (CO), September 6–9, 2015. Abstract 943.
69. Mitsudomi T, Tsai C, Shepherd F, et al. AZD9291 in pre-treated T790M positive advanced NSCLC: AURA2 phase II study [abstract]. Presented at the 16th World Conference on Lung Cancer. Denver (CO), September 6–9, 2015. Abstract 1406.
70. Ramalingam SS, Yang JCH, Lee CK, et al. AZD9291 in treatment-naïve EGFRm advanced NSCLC: AURA first-line cohort. [Oral presentation]. Presented at the 16th World Conference on Lung Cancer. Denver (CO), September 6–9, 2015. Abstract 1232.
71. Odomzo (sonidegib) [package insert]. East Hanover, NJ: Novartis Pharmaceuticals Corporation; 2015.
72. Migden MR, Guminski A, Gutzmer R, et al. Treatment with two different doses of sonidegib in patients with locally advanced or metastatic basal cell carcinoma (BOLT): a multicentre, randomised, double-blind phase 2 trial. Lancet Oncol 2015;16(6):716–28.
73. Erivedge (vismodegib) [package insert]. South San Francisco, CA: Genentech USA; 2015.

Human Papillomavirus–Associated Oropharyngeal Squamous Cell Carcinoma: A Review

Elizabeth M. Garland, MPAS, PA-C*, Lauren C. Parker, MPAS, PA-C, RD

KEYWORDS

- HPV • Human papillomavirus • Oropharynx cancer
- Oropharyngeal squamous carcinoma • HPV vaccination

KEY POINTS

- Nontender unilateral neck masses present in patients aged 40 to 60, especially in nonsmoking men, should raise a high clinical suspicion for oropharyngeal squamous carcinoma.
- All tumor arising in the oropharynx should be tested for presence of human papillomavirus (HPV)/p16.
- Early-stage oropharyngeal HPV related cancers can be treated by surgery or radiation, and later-stage HPV oropharynx cancers are treated with a combination of radiation and chemotherapy.
- Consideration to include HPV status in future staging models for oropharyngeal squamous carcinoma.
- Recommendation to vaccinate children ages 9 to 26 with the 3-dose series for prevention of HPV infection.

INTRODUCTION

There are more than 47,000 new cases of head and neck cancer diagnosed each year.[1] With the surgeon general's warning about the risks of tobacco, the rate of head and neck cancer declined significantly, but a rising trend of epidemic proportions of oropharyngeal squamous cell carcinoma (OPSCC) is being seen. Roughly one-third of all head and neck cancers are identified as being located in the oropharynx, which includes the soft palate, tonsil fossa, base of tongue, and posterior pharyngeal wall.[1] The most common cause of all head and neck cancer is a synergistic relationship of tobacco and alcohol use.[2] Even though there has been a dramatic decrease in tobacco use over the past 50 years, rates of oropharyngeal cancer are increasing.

Disclosure Statement: The authors have nothing to disclose.
Department of Head and Neck Surgery, University of Texas MD Anderson Cancer Center, 1515 Holcombe Boulevard, Unit 1445, Houston, TX 77030, USA
* Corresponding author.
E-mail address: emgarland@mdanderson.org

Physician Assist Clin 1 (2016) 465–477
http://dx.doi.org/10.1016/j.cpha.2016.03.010   physicianassistant.theclinics.com
2405-7991/16/$ – see front matter Published by Elsevier Inc.

Further investigation into the etiology of these malignancies has revealed a strong association with the human papillomavirus (HPV). Incidence rates and current trend in decreasing tobacco use are depicted in **Fig. 1**.

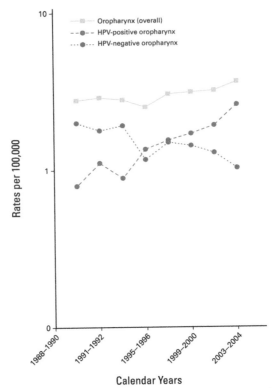

Calendar Years

Trends in Current Cigarette Smoking by High School Students[a] and Adults[b] — United States, 1965–2014

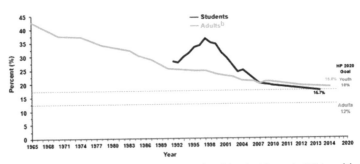

Fig. 1. Graphs show the down-trend in smoking with a rising incidence in HPV-positive oropharyngeal cancer. [a] Percentage of high students who smoked cigarettes on 1 or more of the 30 days preceding the survey (Youth Risk Behavior Survey, 1991–2013). [b] Percentage of adult who are cigarettes smokers (National Health Interview Survey, 1965–2014). (*From* Centers for Disease Control and Prevention (CDC). Trends in current cigarette smoking among high school students and adults, United States, 1965–2011. Available at: http://www.cdc.gov/tobacco/data_statistics/tables/trends/cig_smoking/. Accessed November 14, 2013; and Chaturvedi AK, Engels EA, Pfeiffer RM, et al: Human papillomavirus and rising oropharyngeal cancer incidence in the United States. J Clin Oncol 2011;29:4294–301.)

HPV is a nonenveloped, double-stranded DNA virus with an affinity for the epithelial layer of mucosa (**Fig. 2**).

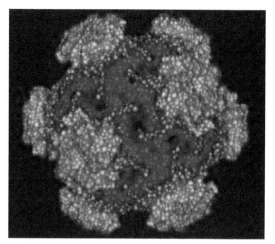

Fig. 2. A computer-rendered representation of the HPV virus. (*From* Mehanna H, Jones TM, Gregoire V, et al. Oropharyngeal carcinoma related to human papillomavirus. BMJ 2010;340(7752):880; with permission.)

The virus is sexually transmitted, and it is hypothesized that the sexual revolution of the middle twentieth century contributed in large part to its prominence. It is the most common sexually transmitted infection in the United States with 14 million new cases each year.[3] Most patients that are infected are symptom-free, and 90% of infections resolve spontaneously within 2 years. Rates of infection continue to increase due to a combination of factors, including lack of education regarding the vaccination and lack of screening (**Fig. 3**).

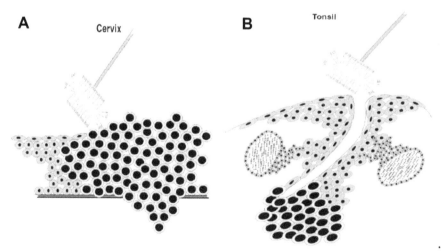

Fig. 3. (*A*) Cervical brushing technique to collect cells for HPV screening. (*B*) Deep tonsil crypts preventing access by brush collection of cells for HPV screening. (*From* Lingen MW. Brush-based cytology screening in the tonsils and cervix: there is a difference! Cancer Prev Res (Phila) 2011;4(9):1351; with permission.)

There are greater than 100 different genotypes, including types 6 and 11, which are responsible for 90% of genital warts, and types 16 and 18, which account for the development of cervical, anal, and oropharyngeal cancer. Strain 16 has the strongest predilection for oropharyngeal cancer and accounts for 85% to 90% of HPV-positive OPSCC.[4] These 4 genotypes are included in the quadrivalent HPV vaccine, recommended for routine use in girls and boys between the ages of 11 and 12.[5]

For HPV-related tumors, the carcinogenic process begins with the inactivation of tumor supressors by oncoproteins. The 2 high-risk oncoproteins, E7 and E6, inactivate the tumor suppressor protein 53 (p53) and retinoblastoma (Rb) tumor suppressor. Deficiency of p53 and Rb leads to physiologic cell death and an elimination of cell-cycle checkpoints; this allows for uninhibited progression of the virus through the cell cycle and genomic integration in the affected cells. Even though the virus is cleared by the immune system, the genetically altered cells are maintained in the mucosal lining.[6] It is unknown why some patients clear the virus entirely without permanent cell disruption whereas others retain the viral DNA within their cells.

HPV-positive oropharyngeal carcinoma is commonly seen in the Caucasian male population in the fourth and fifth decades of life.[7] Patients tend to have a larger number of sexual partners, particularly oral sex partners.[6] It is postulated that the viral load of infected cervical tissue is greater than penile tissue, leading to the increase rate of carcinoma in men. Furthermore, HPV-positive oropharyngeal carcinoma is more common among patients of higher socioeconomic status and education.[7] The HPV-positive patient tends to be a never smoker with minimal history of alcohol consumption and few other comorbidities (**Box 1**).

Box 1
Risk factors for oropharyngeal cancer

- Male gender
- Aged 40 to 60
- High socioeconomic status
- Never smoker
- High number of sexual partners/oral sex partners

The most likely presentation is a nontender neck mass. There may be some associated otalgia, dysphagia, or odynophagia, but it is generally asymptomatic. Because of the nonspecific symptoms, patients often present with locoregionally advanced stage disease. Despite this, patients diagnosed with HPV-positive OPSCC have a better prognosis than HPV-negative carcinomas.[8] When a patient presents with concerning signs and symptoms, in addition to a medical and social history similar to that listed above, a thorough head and neck examination is essential. The proximal oropharynx may be directly visualized, including visualization of the upper aerodigestive tract by indirect mirror examination, and more optimally, a flexible nasopharyngolaryngoscope (**Fig. 4**). Palpation of the neck and oropharynx is essential, because it may reveal submucosal or deep cervical masses that cannot be visualized.

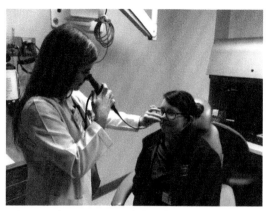

Fig. 4. Flexible nasopharyngolaryngoscopy of the pharynx.

DIAGNOSIS

In the outpatient primary care setting or urgent care setting, a conservative treatment with a course of broad spectrum antibiotics to resolve infectious or reactive lymphade-nopathy is reasonable. If symptoms such as: sore throat, neck mass, ear or jaw pain, or pain with swallowing persists after conservative management, referral for evaluation by an otolaryngologist (ENT) and cross-sectional imaging is recommended (**Fig. 5**).

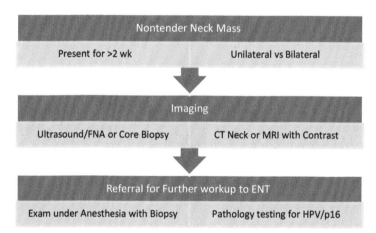

Fig. 5. Flow chart representing typical workup for patient with a neck mass.

Diagnostic workup includes tissue diagnosis with biopsy of the neck mass by ultrasound-guided fine-needle aspiration (FNA) or core biopsy (**Fig. 6**). FNA is a safe, widely available technique that provides tissue for diagnosis and may help some patients avoid general anesthesia for diagnosis.

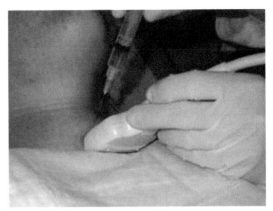

Fig. 6. Ultrasound-guided FNA of a neck mass. (Available at: http://endocrinediseases.org/thyroid/img/pic_fna_nodule.jpg. Accessed January 21, 2016.)

HPV and p16 biomarkers are standard of care testing for pathology specimens, but may need to be requested individually, depending on the laboratory. Cross-sectional imaging for staging and diagnosis, computed tomography (CT) neck with contrast, or MRI of the head and neck with contrast are adequate for demonstrating abnormalities in these areas. A cystic neck mass seen on CT scan or MRI is characteristic of an HPV-related squamous carcinoma in the oropharynx.[6] PET scanning is not recommended for initial locoregional screening in patients unless other testing fails to reveal a primary site or adverse features are found on imaging, such as N2c-N3 neck disease or lung abnormalities on cross-sectional imaging, which may indicate distant metastasis. Most patients should undergo diagnostic endoscopy by examination under general anesthesia (EUA) with directed biopsies of the nasopharynx, oropharynx, hypopharynx, and larynx to establish the primary tumor site. If surgical management

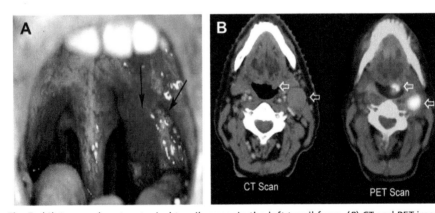

Fig. 7. (A) Arrows denote a typical tonsil cancer in the left tonsil fossa. (B) CT and PET image of a left tonsil tumor denoted by the medial arrow and ipsilateral neck lymph node metastasis denoted by the lateral arrow. (*From* Flint P, Haughey B, Lund V, et al, editors. Cummings otolaryngology head and neck surgery. 6th edition. Philadelphia: Elsevier; and About cancer. PET and CT scans of head and neck cancers. Available at: http://www.aboutcancer.com/throat_anatomy_pet.htm. Accessed January 21, 2016, with permission.)

is being considered for the patient, EUA can also provide critical information about respectability, such as how lateralized the disease is in the tonsil or base of tongue, amount of extension of the disease to adjacent structures, patient's ability to open their mouth, and ease of exposure of the target tissues for surgical therapy with neck extension and mouth opening.

Once pathology has been obtained of the primary oropharyngeal disease or neck disease, the current recommendation is to test all cancers for the presence of HPV.[6] The surrogate markers for HPV in pathologic tissue can be tested for by the presence of p16 through immunohistochemistry on pathologic testing[6,9] (**Fig. 7**).

STAGING AND DIAGNOSIS

The American Joint Commission on Cancer staging model, currently in the 7th edition, is most often used to classify TNM staging for oropharyngeal squamous carcinoma.

A characteristic of HPV-related oropharyngeal squamous carcinoma is a small primary with multiple lymph nodes. HPV-associated oropharyngeal cancer most commonly presents as T1-T2-sized tumor and N1-N3 neck disease with N2 nodal staging as the dominant stage[6,10] (**Figs. 8** and **9**).

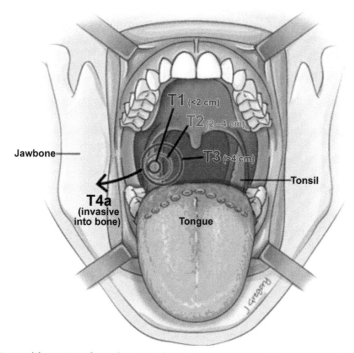

Fig. 8. Tumor (T) staging of oropharyngeal squamous carcinoma. T1, tumor less than 2 cm; T2, tumor 2 cm up to 4 cm; T3, tumor more than 4 cm; T4, tumor invading structures: mandible, extrinsic muscles of the tongue, or hyoid bone. (*From* Head Neck and Cancer Guide. Determining the stage of the cancer. Available at: http://www.headandneckcancerguide.org/adults/introduction-to-head-and-neck-cancer/throat-cancer/oropharyngeal-cancer/tonsil-cancer/stage-cancer/. Accessed January 21, 2016.)

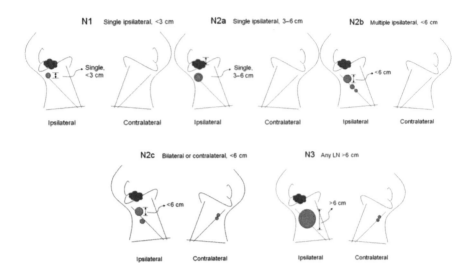

Fig. 9. Staging of neck metastases in oropharyngeal squamous carcinoma. N0, no clinically palpable lymphadenopathy, no adenopathy on imaging; N1, a single lymph node metastasis less than 3 cm; N2a, a single lymph node measuring 3 to 6 cm ipsilateral to the primary site; N2b, multiple lymph nodes ipsilateral to the primary tumor or matted lymph nodes; N2c, multiple lymph nodes ipsilateral and contralateral to the primary tumor; N3, any lymph node metastasis greater than 6 cm in its greatest dimension. (*From* Oral cancer: investigations and stage. Available at: http://www.intelligentdental.com/2012/02/28/oral-cancer-investigations-and-staging/. Accessed January 21, 2016.)

MULTIDISCIPLINARY TREATMENT TEAM

Patients that present with oropharyngeal squamous carcinoma should have multidisciplinary evaluation including an ENT specialist or head and neck surgeon, medical oncology, and radiation oncology. Additional evaluation by the dental and speech therapy teams will be necessary to assess the dentition as well as swallowing function before treatment begins. If patients have the resources for treatment at an academic center, then this is optimal for access to clinical trials and multidisciplinary evaluation. Physician assistants (PA) are an integral part of the team with a role in providing support for diagnostic workup, education, and treatment planning. The treatment team for each discipline includes a physician, advanced practice provider, nurse, and scheduler to ensure continuity of care in treatment and surveillance. PAs and other advanced practice providers lead the head and neck survivorship program at the authors' center to continue annual monitoring of patients that have completed 2 years surveillance from their last treatment.

TREATMENT

Treatment selection for patients with HPV-related oropharyngeal cancer is based on patient comorbidities, performance status, tumor location in selection of surgical and nonsurgical approaches, and staging.[11] The ultimate goal of treatment is at the intersection to optimize disease control, decrease toxicity and morbidity of treatment, and maintain quality of life and functional status.[6] The most common treatment side effects for oropharyngeal carcinoma relate to speech and swallowing. Ultimately, HPV association shows increased survival and response to treatment regardless of choice of treatment modality with high cure rates for patients.[6,11] Patients can be counseled on swallowing exercises and jaw exercises to maintain function of the swallow during treatment and prevent aspiration. Dental extractions should be considered before any radiation-based treatment to prevent osteoradionecrosis of the mandible, as well as counseling on the post-treatment effects of radiation, and need for fluoride treatment.

Historically, surgical treatment in the oropharynx required large cosmetically averse surgery that involved cutting the mandible to access the oropharynx and large flap reconstruction with devastating effects to swallowing and cosmetic appearance. Pathology usually revealed multiple adverse features such as positive margins, perineural invasion, and multilevel positive lymphadenopathy invariably requiring postoperative multimodality treatment with chemoradiation.[9] Patients often had significant post-treatment toxicity, such as trismus, dysphagia, and laryngeal dysfunction after multimodality treatment with surgery, chemotherapy, and radiation. Often, patients required permanent feeding tube placement or tracheostomy placement. To reduce treatment, morbidity, and dysfunction, a paradigm shift was made to treating patients with concurrent radiation and chemotherapy, because these treatments proved to produce good overall survival and disease control. This treatment protocol has been the mainstay of oropharyngeal cancer treatment from 1985 to 2001.[10] However, advances in minimally invasive techniques, such as the robotic surgery system, allow surgeons a transoral approach for primary surgery. In appropriate patients, these advanced techniques allow radiation to be given in a reduced dose, or chemotherapy and radiation avoided altogether. Current radiation treatment is delivered with intensity-modulated radiation therapy (IMRT) to delivery precise doses for treatment while sparing important functional organs in the head and neck[9] (**Box 2**).

Early-Stage Treatment

Stage I/II disease with small primary tumor and low-volume neck disease can be treated with a surgical approach versus IMRT radiation alone. Small T1-T2-sized tumors located in the base of tongue, tonsil, glossopharyngeal sulcus, and lateral pharyngeal wall are best suited for evaluation for a surgical approach. IMRT radiation alone also works well for early-stage disease. Transoral surgery shows a 91% local control at 2 years and overall survival of 91%.[9]

Given HPV oropharyngeal cancer's improved prognosis with any treatment modality, current trials look to answer if traditional radiation dosing for treatment could be de-escalated. Studies have shown that patients that are favorable surgical candidates show no significant difference in prognosis and survival between surgical treatment and nonsurgical treatment for HPV-positive oropharyngeal carcinoma.[10,11] Surgery can be performed for selected patients with adjuvant radiation therapy for adverse features, such as positive margins, perineural invasion, lymphovascular invasion, or upstaging features, such as microscopic disease in multiple positive nodes, or upstaging with extracapsular extension.

Advanced Stage Treatment

Patients that present with advanced stage disease are typically not surgical candidates and will require multiple modality treatment with chemotherapy and radiation. Patients presenting with T1-T3 tumors with N2b neck disease can be considered for concurrent chemotherapy and radiation therapy. Patients with bilateral neck disease and bulky neck disease may be considered for neoadjuvant/induction chemotherapy to reduce the tumor burden before concurrent chemotherapy and radiation therapy.[6,9,11] Most patients present in stage III/IV and are treated with concurrent chemotherapy and radiation therapy. Current trials are looking at targeted agents, such as cetuximab (Erbitux), to see if these agents can be used to reduce toxicity associated with chemotherapy.

Box 2
Example of treatment modalities based on staging

T1-T2, N0-N1	Transoral surgery vs radiation alone
T1-T2, N2a	Transoral surgery vs radiation alone
T1-T4, N2b	Radiation and chemotherapy, concurrently
Any T, N2c-N3	Induction chemotherapy followed by radiation and chemotherapy

---

PROGNOSIS

Squamous carcinoma of the oropharynx that is caused by HPV has an excellent prognosis with a survival rate of 80% to 90% at 5 years despite late-stage III/IV diagnosis and increasing incidence in the population.[6] The association with the HPV virus confers sensitivity to treatment with progression-free survival and has been independently shown as the strongest prognostic factor in predicting survival and locoregional control in patients with HPV-positive OPSCC.[6,12] Factors affecting prognosis in patients with oropharyngeal squamous carcinoma are HPV status, tobacco use status, tumor stage, and nodal staging.[13] Patients that are HPV-negative and are currently smoking with high T stage and N stage have a poorer prognosis than patients who are HPV positive and have never smoked. HPV-positive oropharyngeal SCC patients diagnosed at an advanced stage (stage III/IV) have a better response to treatment and have better progression free survival than patients with HPV-negative oropharyngeal SCC (**Fig. 10**).[8,10,14]

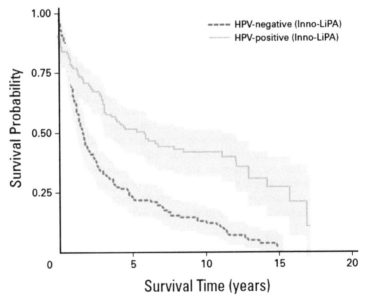

Fig. 10. Survival in patients with HPV-positive versus HPV-negative OPSCC as determined by Inno-LiPA assay for HPV genotyping. (*From* Chaturvedi AK, Engels EA, Pfeiffer RM, et al. Human papillomavirus and rising oropharyngeal cancer incidence in the United States. J Clin Oncol 2011;29:4298; with permission.)

Current studies have proposed that the HPV-positive oropharynx tumors may be more biologically responsive to therapy, explaining the overall survival rate of HPV-related oropharynx cancer without significant change in treatment protocol.[15] Patients with HPV-positive disease who also smoke show less reliability on HPV as a good prognostic indicator because tobacco use may alter the behavior of HPV-related oropharynx cancer and could alter response to treatment. Tobacco use in the patient with HPV-positive oropharynx cancer could present a confounding variable for predicting treatment outcomes and survival.[6] Cancer has a high rate of locoregional control but does not offer protection in reducing risk for distant metastatic disease[15] (see **Fig. 10**).

SURVEILLANCE

At completion of treatment, it is recommended for posttreatment patients to continue contact with their treating teams with a quarterly surveillance approach of directed physical examination, cross-sectional imaging, and symptom-based management of posttreatment side effects. Side effects from radiation can include dry mouth, dysphagia, and osteoradionecrosis. A typical follow-up schedule is quarterly for the first year after completing treatment with cross-sectional imaging and thyroid function testing. Thyroid function is followed closely because hypothyroidism is common after external beam radiation to the neck with direct effect on the thyroid. Patients are examined every 4 months through year 2 after completion of treatment. Patients are followed annually until 5 years after completion of treatment. After 2 years with no evidence of disease, patients are eligible to be transitioned to the head and neck survivorship program, wherein patients continue under surveillance with cross-sectional imaging.

PREVENTION

HPV infection and ultimately HPV-related cancer can be prevented through vaccination.[12,16] There is no screening for detecting oropharyngeal cancer, so vaccination for prevention is paramount.[17] There is no current recommendation for HPV vaccination in sexually active adults. There are currently 2 US Food and Drug Administration (FDA) -approved vaccines for prevention of HPV infection. Both vaccines are approved for use in male and female patients aged 9 to 26. Gardasil, a quadrivalent vaccine, was FDA approved in 2006 for prevention of infection by serotypes 6, 11, 16, and 18. Bivalent vaccine, Cervarix, was FDA approved in 2009 for prevention of infection by high-risk serotypes 16 and 18 only. Each vaccine is given in a 3-dose series at 0 months, 2 months, and 6 months. It is recommended to be given before initiation of any sexual behaviors for maximum efficacy.[18] Current vaccination statistics show that despite published recommendation for vaccination, only one-third to one-half of eligible girls and young women completed the 3-dose vaccine series. The most commonly cited reason for lack of vaccination by patients was a lack of recommendation for the vaccine by providers, and the most common reason for providers to not recommend the vaccination were due to discussing sexual behavior with young patients and parents as well as lack of reimbursement for vaccine.[16]

DISCUSSION

HPV-related oropharyngeal squamous carcinoma has an excellent prognosis, high response to therapy, high curability, and disease-free survival, suggesting that HPV-positive oropharynx cancer is a disease separate from HPV-negative oropharynx cancer.[11] The current TNM staging model does not adequately represent the good prognosis of HPV-related oropharynx cancer. Several studies have proposed the inclusion of HPV status in staging to represent improved prognosis related to HPV-positive disease.[10] It is extrapolated that if current trends of HPV-positive oropharyngeal squamous carcinoma continue, HPV-positive OPSCC will make up the majority of cancers to the head and neck in the United States in the next 20 years. This projection demonstrates the need for increased vaccination in young populations for prevention.[12]

With good prognosis and high survival rates in younger cancer populations aged 40 to 60, patients will have long-term side effects from treatment such as dysphagia and swallowing difficulty. Radiation and chemoradiation therapy have an increased risk of delayed toxicity with dysphagia and aspiration being the most significant latent toxicities affecting the function of the swallow and quality of life for patients.[9] Some patients require life-long need for tube feeding secondary to aspiration and tracheostomy for airway protection, and in severe cases, patients will require laryngectomy to manage laryngeal dysfunction and aspiration. Current studies aim to answer the question of de-escalated therapies, such as transoral surgical resection, targeted chemotherapy agents, reduced radiation doses, and altered radiation fractionation to reduce morbidity and latent toxicity while maintaining high cure rate and disease control.

In closing, the increase in HPV-related oropharynx cancer highlights the need to increase awareness of the epidemic of HPV-related oropharynx cancer to identify patients at an early stage and refer for further evaluation, management, and treatment as well as raise awareness for increased vaccination in young populations for prevention of HPV-related cancers.

ACKNOWLEDGMENTS

The authors would like to thank Amy Hessel, MD, FACS, for her assistance and collaboration.

REFERENCES

1. Siegel R, Miller K, Jermal A. Cancer statistics, 2015. CA Cancer J Clin 2010;65:5–29.
2. Sturgis EM, Cinciripini PM. Trends in head and neck cancer incidence in relation to smoking prevalence: an emerging epidemic of human papillomavirus-associated cancers? Cancer 2007;110(7):1429–35.
3. Gayar OH, Ruterbusch JJ, Elshaikh M, et al. Oropharyngeal carcinoma in young adults: an alarming national trend. Otolaryngol Head Neck Surg 2014;150(4):594–601.
4. D'Souza G, Kreimer AR, Viscidi R, et al. Case-control study of human papilloma virus and oropharyngeal cancer. N Engl J Med 2007;356:1944–56.
5. Centers for Disease Control and Prevention (CDC). Sexually transmitted diseases surveillance. Available at: http://www.cdc.gov/std/stats14/other.htm#hpv. Accessed November 17, 2015.
6. Ang KK, Sturgis EM. Human papillomavirus as a marker of the natural history and response to therapy of head and neck squamous cell carcinoma. Semin Radiat Oncol 2012;22(2):128–42.
7. Dahlstrom KR, Bell D, Hanby D, et al. Socioeconomic characteristics of patients with oropharyngeal carcinoma according to tumor HPV status, patient smoking status, and sexual behavior. Oral Oncol 2015;51(9):832–8.
8. Dahlstrom KR, Anderson KS, Cheng JN, et al. HPV serum antibodies as predictors of survival and disease progression in patients with HPV-positive squamous cell carcinoma of the oropharynx. Clin Cancer Res 2015;21(12):2861–9.

9. Holsinger FC, Ferris RL. Transoral endoscopic head and neck surgery and its role within the multidisciplinary treatment paradigm of oropharynx cancer: robotics, lasers, and clinic trials. J Clin Oncol 2015;33:3285–92.
10. Dahlstrom KR, Calzada G, Hanby JD, et al. An evolution in demographics, treatment, and outcomes of oropharyngeal cancer at a major cancer center. Cancer 2013;119:81–9.
11. Salazar CR, Smith RV, Garg MK, et al. Human papillomavirus-associated head and neck squamous cell carcinoma survival: a comparison by tumor site and initial treatment. Head Neck Pathol 2014;8:77–87.
12. Chaturvedi AK, Engels EA, Pfeiffer RM, et al. Human papillomavirus and rising oropharyngeal cancer incidence in the United States. J Clin Oncol 2011;29: 4294–301.
13. Ang KK, Harris J, Wheeler R, et al. Human papillomavirus and survival of patients with oropharyngeal cancer. N Engl J Med 2010;363:24–35.
14. Mehanna H, Jones TM, Gregoire V, et al. Oropharyngeal carcinoma related to human papillomavirus. BMJ 2010;340:c1439.
15. Fakhry C, Zhang Q, Nguyen-Tan PF, et al. Human papillomavirus and overall survival after progression of oropharyngeal squamous cell carcinoma. J Clin Oncol 2014;32:3365–73.
16. Jemal A, Simard EP, Dorell C, et al. Annual report to the nation on the status of cancer, 1975-2009, featuring the burden and trends in human papillomavirus (HPV)-associated cancers and HPV vaccination coverage levels. J Natl Cancer Inst 2013;105:175–201.
17. Anderson KS, Dahlstrom KR, Cheng JA, et al. HPV16 antibodies as risk factors for oropharyngeal cancer and their association with tumor HPV and smoking status. Oral Oncol 2015;51:662–7.
18. D'Souza G, Dempsey A. The role of HPV in head and neck cancer and review of the HPV vaccine. Prev Med 2011;53:S5–11.

Ovarian Cancer: Practice Essentials

Kristine Prazak, PA-C, MS[a],*, Jessica Gahres, PA-C, MS[b]

KEYWORDS

- Ovarian cancer • Surgical debulking • Chemotherapy • BRCA1 • BRCA2
- Bevacizumab • PARP inhibitors • Immunotherapy

KEY POINTS

- The initial presentation for ovarian cancer can be subtle and it is important for physician assistants to recognize symptoms.
- Treatment consists of surgical debulking followed by chemotherapy.
- New research efforts on treatment continue to be developed and include immunotherapy.

INTRODUCTION

Ms Smith is a 60-year-old woman who presented to her primary care physician with concerns of intermittent pelvic pain along with dysuria for the past few months. She was treated for a urinary tract infection. The patient's symptoms did not improve on antibiotics and she then followed up with her gynecologist. On bimanual pelvic examination, the patient was found to have an irregular mass that was palpated in the right lower quadrant. Ms Smith was then sent for a pelvic ultrasound that identified a right ovarian multiseptated cystic mass with severe nodular thickening suspicious for malignancy. A computed tomography scan of the abdomen and pelvis revealed a complex mass in the right cul-de-sac and omental masses. Serum cancer antigen (CA)-125 testing was sent and resulted as 317 µ/mL (normal < 35 µ/mL). What is the most likely diagnosis?

Differential: Dermoid cyst, uterine myoma, ovarian malignancy, follicular cyst.

DISCUSSION

Ovarian cancer is the second most common and the most deadly gynecologic malignancy in the United States. The 5-year survival for a diagnosis of ovarian cancer is on average 45.6%.[1] Five-year survival rates for patients diagnosed with stage I disease

Disclosures: None.
[a] Department of Physician Assistant Studies, New York Institute of Technology, Old Westbury, NY, USA; [b] Department of Medicine, Gynecologic Medical Oncology, Memorial Sloan Kettering Cancer Center, New York, NY, USA
* Corresponding author. Northern Boulevard, P.O. Box 8000, Old Westbury, NY 11568-8000.
E-mail address: kprazak@nyit.edu

Physician Assist Clin 1 (2016) 479–487
http://dx.doi.org/10.1016/j.cpha.2016.03.009
physicianassistant.theclinics.com

are close to 90%. However, approximately 75% of women are diagnosed with advanced stage disease (stage III or IV). As the stage of disease advances, the survival rate decreases dramatically. For example, the most recent data reported by the National Cancer Institute shows that those women diagnosed with stage IV disease have a 5-year survival rate of 17%[2] (**Fig. 1**).

A woman's lifetime risk of developing ovarian cancer is 1.3%. Women with a family history of ovarian cancer have an increased risk.[1] The risk factors for ovarian cancer include advanced age (ovarian cancer is most frequently diagnosed among women aged 55–64),[1] nulliparity, primary infertility, hormone therapy, obesity, and a family history of 2 or more first-degree relatives with ovarian cancer.

Mutations in the *BRCA1* or *2* genes are associated with hereditary breast and ovarian cancer syndromes, and can be associated with early onset disease, accounting for approximately 15% of ovarian carcinomas.[3] The lifetime ovarian cancer risk for women with a *BRCA1* mutation is estimated to be between 35% and 70%. This means that if 100 women had a *BRCA1* mutation, between 35 and 70 of them would develop ovarian cancer. For women with *BRCA2* mutations, the risk has been estimated to be between 10% and 30% by age 70. These mutations also increase the risks for primary peritoneal carcinoma and fallopian tube carcinoma. The lifetime risk of ovarian cancer also increases by about 10% in women with hereditary nonpolyposis colon cancer.[4]

There are certain factors that are thought to be protective; these include: younger age at pregnancy and first birth (≤25 years at pregnancy and first birth confers 30%-60% reduced risk), breast feeding, oral contraception (5-year cumulative use of oral contraceptive pills decreases lifetime risk by one-half), prophylactic salpingo-oophrectomy in high risk women, and bilateral tubal ligation. It is estimated that the risk of ovarian and fallopian tube cancer can be reduced by 80% for *BRCA1* and *BRCA2* mutation carriers who undergo a prophylactic oophorectomy.[5] The American College of Obstetricians and Gynecologists recommends that risk-reducing salpingo-oophorectomy be offered by age 40 years for women with *BRCA1* or *BRCA2* mutations.[6,7]

Ovarian cancer is often thought of as a "silent killer." The symptoms of ovarian cancer tend to be nonspecific and are confused with gastrointestinal, urologic, or other conditions. A study published in 2000 by Goff and colleagues[8] surveyed 1725 women with a diagnosis of ovarian cancer. When asked if they had symptoms before diagnosis, 77% reported abdominal symptoms, 70% gastrointestinal, 58% pain, 50% constitutional, 34% urinary, and 26% pelvic. Only 11% of women with stage I or II disease and 3% with stage III or IV disease reported no symptoms before their diagnosis.

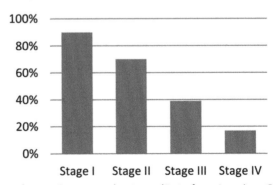

Fig. 1. Survival rates for ovarian cancer, by stage. (*Data from* American Cancer Society. Survival rates for ovarian cancer, by stage. Available at: www.cancer.org/cancer/ovariancancer/detailedguide/ovarian-cancer-survival-rates. Accessed April 18, 2016.)

A thorough medical history is important and can offer clues that lead to early diagnosis. Symptoms that are new in onset, occur almost daily, and are more severe than expected should raise red flags in this age group and prompt the clinician to investigate further. In 2007, the Gynecologic Cancer Foundation, American Cancer Society, and Society of Gynecologic Oncology issued a consensus statement on early symptoms. Supportive studies have shown that the symptoms of bloating, pelvic or abdominal pain, difficulty eating or feeling full quickly, and urinary symptoms (urgency or frequency) are more likely to occur in women with ovarian cancer than in the general public. A prospective case-control study of women who visited 2 primary care clinics was compared with women who presented preoperatively with a pelvic mass (84 benign, 44 malignant) noted that ovarian cancer symptoms are more likely to be progressive, persistent, frequent (20–30 times a month), more severe, and multiple. For example, the median number of symptoms among women with ovarian cancer was 8 compared with a 4 in a primary clinic population. The number of recurring symptoms was 4 compared with 2, respectively.[9,10]

Diagnosis

In women presenting with symptoms associated with ovarian cancer, initial evaluation should include a thorough history and physical examination, including pelvic and rectal examinations. Any abnormal findings should then be referred for transvaginal ultrasound examination and serum tumor marker CA-125. CA-125 is a protein that is found on ovarian cancer cells. This test is useful if it is elevated when the cancer is first diagnosed. It can be used to see if the cancer is responding to treatment by seeing a decrease in levels. In a woman who has ovarian cancer, an increase in CA-125 can mean that the cancer has progressed or recurred.

Women diagnosed with ovarian cancer usually present with symptoms at advanced stage disease (stage III or IV) and symptoms can be acute or subacute. Acute symptoms, such as pleural effusion or bowel obstruction, require urgent care. Subacute symptoms, such as weight gain, pelvic pain, adnexal mass, or gastrointestinal symptoms, usually can be evaluated in an outpatient setting. The finding of an adnexal mass on pelvic examination or on imaging is the most common presentation of ovarian cancer. The American College of Obstetrics and Gynecologists recommends that all women with a mass suspicious for cancer to be referred to a gynecologic oncologist for further evaluation.[11]

There are several factors that can lead to delays in diagnosis. Some are patient related, such as attributing the symptoms to other factors that can include menstrual irregularities, menopause, aging, pregnancy, and stress. On average, women wait 2 to 3 months after symptom onset to seek medical attention. Provider delays occur when women are misdiagnosed initially and treated for another condition. Common conditions include irritable bowel syndrome, stress, gastritis, depression, urinary tract infections, and constipation.[12]

There are no effective screening strategies for early detection of ovarian cancer. Initially the serum tumor marker, and CA-125, along with pelvic ultrasound examinations held promise for early detection of disease. However, results of a large randomized trial of more than 78,000 women found that screening with transvaginal ultrasound examination and CA-125 did not decrease mortality from ovarian cancer.[13] The authors of the study concluded that women at average risk for ovarian cancer should not undergo routine screening. This recommendation was supported by others. Currently, there are no data supporting routine screening for the general population. Routine screening is not recommended by any professional society.[14]

Women in the high-risk category include those with an identified *BRCA* gene mutation and family history of cancer. These women should be referred for genetic counseling. National Comprehensive Cancer Network guidelines recommend risk reducing salpingo-oophorectomy for women with known *BRCA1* or *BRCA2*, typically between the ages of 35 to 40 and upon completion of childbearing. Screening of high-risk women with CA 125 and transvaginal ultrasound examination every 6 months has been practiced; however, there are inconclusive data demonstrating benefits or improved survival rates in this population.[3]

Molecular Pathogenesis

Epithelial ovarian carcinoma is the most common histologic type of cancer involving the ovary, fallopian tube, or peritoneum. It consists of a heterogenous group of neoplasms that can be divided further into separate histologic subtypes; high-grade serous (70%–80%), endometrioid carcinoma (10%), clear cell carcinomas (10%), mucinous carcinoma (3%), and low-grade serous carcinoma (<5%). The most common presentation of epithelial ovarian cancer is high-grade serous.[15] Other, rarer subtypes include transitional cell carcinoma, carcinosarcoma, and undifferentiated carcinoma.

There is distinct morphology and heterogeneity of epithelial ovarian carcinomas that has made it problematic in elucidating the pathogenesis.[16] Tumors are characterized by p53 mutation (>80%) and high-level genetic instability.

Epithelial ovarian cancer was traditionally thought to originate from the ovaries, but newer evidence suggests that these neoplasms may actually originate from the fallopian tubes. Pathology from women undergoing prophylactic risk reducing surgery for *BRCA* mutations has identified precursor lesions in the fimbriated end of fallopian tubes called the serous tubal intraepithelial carcinoma. Serous tubal intraepithelial carcinoma was found to resemble high-grade serous ovarian cancer and has been identified in greater than 60% of non-*BRCA* serous ovarian carcinomas.[17]

Epithelial ovarian cancer most often spreads within the peritoneal cavity with metastasis seen to the diaphragm, the surface of the liver, mesentery, omentum, uterus, and paraaortic and pelvic lymph nodes.

TREATMENT
Surgery

If ovarian cancer is suspected, patients should be referred to a gynecologic oncologic surgeon for evaluation. Initial surgery should be a comprehensive staging laparotomy, including a total abdominal hysterectomy, bilateral salpingo-oophorectomy, omentectomy, pelvic and paraortic lymphadenectomy, and appendectomy.[3] The American Joint Committee on Cancer provides the staging system used after surgical cytoreduction. **Box 1** provides an abbreviated description of the stages of ovarian cancer.

Chemotherapy

After surgical staging and cytoreduction for ovarian cancer, most patients with advanced stage disease receive chemotherapy. This treatment is referred to as adjuvant chemotherapy. Treatment is platinum-based therapy, which is a doublet therapy consisting of a taxane and platinum-based chemotherapy. Platinum-based therapy is classified as an alkylating agent that kills cancer cells by binding to DNA and interfering with cell repair and leading to cell death. Studies have shown that a combination of both a platinum-based chemotherapy and a taxol improves the survival of women with ovarian cancer. There are 3 acceptable means for administering treatment: IV

Box 1
Stages of ovarian cancer

Stage I

In stage I, cancer is found in 1 or both ovaries or fallopian tubes.

Stage II

In stage II, cancer is found in 1 or both ovaries or fallopian tubes and has spread into other areas of the pelvis or primary peritoneal cancer is found within the pelvis.

Stage III

In stage III, cancer is found in 1 or both ovaries or fallopian tubes, or is primary peritoneal cancer, and has spread outside the pelvis to other parts of the abdomen and/or to nearby lymph nodes.

Stage IV

In stage IV, cancer has spread beyond the abdomen to other parts of the body. In stage IVB, the cancer has spread to organs and tissues outside the abdomen, including lymph nodes in the groin.

Adapted from Ovarian Epithelial, Fallopian Tube, and Primary Peritoneal Cancer Treatment–Patient Version (PDQ®)Stages of Ovarian Epithelial, Fallopian Tube, and Primary Peritoneal Cancer. Available at: www.cancer.gov/types/ovarian/patient/ovarian-epithelial-treatment-pdq#link/_130.

---

chemotherapy given every 3 weeks, Intraperitoneal chemotherapy, intravenous dose-dense chemotherapy. Studies have shown that intraperitoneal therapy had the documented the longest median survival and is recommended for women with stage III disease or higher.

Observation is recommended for early stage disease (stage 1A or 1B, grade 1 tumors) because survival is greater than 90% with surgery alone.[18,19]

Common side effects related to chemotherapy include fatigue, alopecia, myelosuppression, neuropathy, and nausea and vomiting. Supportive medication is given to help alleviate symptoms of chemotherapy to allow for less toxicity related to treatment.

For patients who are unable to be considered for upfront surgical debulking, usually because complete cytoreduction is not possible at time of surgery, then it would be appropriate to treat with neoadjuvant chemotherapy. This assessment to not proceed with surgical debulking must be made by a gynecologic surgical oncologist before starting neoadjuvant chemotherapy. Confirmation of disease can be made by a biopsy, fine needle aspiration or a paracentesis.

Women with a new diagnosis of ovarian cancer should be referred for genetic testing because germline mutations of *BRCA1* or *BRCA2* account for 15% of ovarian carcinomas.[20]

Future Treatments

In ovarian cancer, surgery and chemotherapy regimens have been the mainstay of treatment. Despite upfront therapy of surgery and traditional chemotherapy, a large majority of women will develop relapse and require additional therapy. However, newer treatments with exciting new mechanisms of action are being developed as treatment options for patients with recurrent ovarian cancer. Several of these new treatment options are described herein.

Poly adenosine diphosphate-ribose polymerase inhibitors

BRCA1 and *BRCA2* is a tumor suppressor gene normally expressed in breast and other tissue including ovarian. The function of this gene is to help repair damaged

DNA, or destroy cells if DNA cannot be repaired. If there is a *BRCA* mutation and damaged DNA is not repaired properly, it could lead to the risk of development of cancer cells.

Poly adenosine diphosphate-ribose polymerase (PARP) inhibitor is an enzyme that is involved in DNA transcription, cell-cycle regulation, and DNA repair. There has been increasing interest in exploring the benefit of PARP inhibitors in cancer therapeutics. Olaparib, an exemplar of a PARP inhibitor, works by inducing a synthetic lethality in *BRCA1/2*-deficient tumors through the formation of double-stranded DNA breaks that cannot be accurately repaired, which therefore leads to cell death.[20]

There are recent data that suggest that the use of olaparib is active in patients with germline *BRCA1* or *BRCA2* mutations, especially those with platinum-sensitive epithelial ovarian cancer. Specifically, olaparib (AZD2281) has been approved by the Food and Drug Administration in the United States to be used as a monotherapy after progression on at least 3 prior lines of chemotherapy.[20] In a large, randomized trial that included 300 women, when compared with placebo there was a significant improvement of progression free survival of 8 versus 5 months. Those who are *BRCA* negative have a lower response rate than those who have a *BRCA* mutation with use of olaparib.[20] Toxicity to olaparib is low with most common side effects being nausea, fatigue, vomiting, and anemia. Other PARP inhibitors are currently being investigated to determine efficacy and optimal dosing. Phase II and III trials are underway to investigate veliparib, niraparib, and rucaparib.

Immunotherapy for ovarian cancer

There has been growing interest in identifying new modalities and approaches to treating ovarian cancer as an alternative to standard therapy. In past decades, there have been advances in understanding the role of the immunogenicity in cancer. This has opened a door for immunotherapy as a potential treatment option in ovarian carcinoma.[21] Immunotherapeutics is an approach to cancer treatment that uses the immune system to eradicate malignancy.

Immunotherapy for ovarian cancer can be divided into 4 treatment categories: monoclonal antibodies, checkpoint inhibitors and immune modulators, therapeutic vaccines, and adoptive T-cell transfer.

Monoclonal antibodies

Monoclonal antibodies target specific antigens on tumor cells. Bevacizumab is a monoclonal antibody that binds to vascular endothelial growth factor, which prevents it from binding to its growth receptor. Blockade of this receptor inhibits growth of tumor-associated blood vessels. This monoclonal antibody has been approved by the US Food and Drug Administration for the treatment of ovarian cancer. Bevacizumab can be used in the setting of recurrent disease, but the role and benefit of bevacizumab in adjuvant treatment is being investigated currently. The National Comprehensive Cancer Network guidelines encourage the participation in ongoing trials to further investigate the role of antiangiogenesis in the treatment of ovarian cancer in both upfront and recurrent settings.

Checkpoint inhibitors and immune modulators

Immune checkpoints, under normal physiologic conditions, are in place to protect tissue from damage when the immune system is responding to an infection. Immune checkpoint proteins can be dysregulated by tumors as an immune resistance mechanism. The blockade of immune checkpoints has opened the possibility for potential antitumor immune therapy in cancer therapeutics.[22]

One important immune checkpoint receptor is the cytotoxic T-lymphocyte associated antigen 4, which is responsible for down modulating amplitude of T-cell activation. In mouse models for sarcoma and colon cancer with use of anti–cytotoxic T-lymphocyte associated antigen 4 antibody it was seen to have antitumor effect.[23] Ipilimumab, an anti–CTLA-4 antibody, has been the first immune checkpoint inhibitor to be approved based on its ability to prolong survival in patients with metastatic melanoma.

Another potential target for immunotherapy is programmed cell death 1, which is a transmembrane protein expressed on T cells, B cells, and natural killer cells. It is an inhibitory molecule that binds to programmed cell death–ligand 1 and is expressed on multiple tissue types including many tumor cells. When activated, it directly inhibits apoptosis of tumor cells. Inhibiting programmed cell death 1 antibodies, such as nivolumab and pembrolizumab, have been shown to prolong overall survival in randomized trials in metastatic melanoma.

Both cytotoxic T-lymphocyte associated antigen 4 and programmed cell death 1 are being studied in clinical trials for use in the recurrent setting for ovarian cancer. There is hope that the same mechanism of action and efficacy can be translated to ovarian cancer treatment.

Therapeutic vaccines
Researchers have identified specific cancer-associated antigens, which are only expressed on cancer cells and not healthy tissue, that would elicit a response from the immune system to destroy cancer cells. Therapeutic vaccines aim to use the immune system to "attack" tumor cells by targeting specifically cancer associated antigens.[24] Currently, phase I and II clinical trials are open at various institutes and are actively recruiting patients.

Adoptive T-cell transfer
In adoptive T-cell transfer, the patient's T cells are collected through apheresis and the T cells are then modified chemically to enhance their behavior. Patients are given a short course of chemotherapy and the activated immune cells are infused back into the patient with the goal of improving the patient's immune system. This mechanism has been most extensively studied in hematologic malignancies and has shown success in B-cell acute lymphoblastic leukemia.[25]

There are several phase I and II trials ongoing to test engineered T cells in patients with ovarian cancer.

SUMMARY

Ms Smith met with a gynecologic oncology surgeon and underwent complete surgical debulking with final pathology showing stage IIIC high-grade serous ovarian carcinoma. The patient received adjuvant chemotherapy and completed 6 cycles of intravenous/intraperitoneal paclitaxel (Taxol) and cisplatin. Response to treatment was evaluated by computed tomography scan of the chest, abdomen, and pelvis, which was negative for malignancy. The CA-125 fell from 317 μ/mL at diagnosis to 7 μ/mL (normal, <35 μ/mL) after treatment. Ms Smith is considered to have a "complete response" with a normal clinical examination, negative CA-125, and no evidence of cancer on her computed tomography scan. The patient was then seen every 3 months for surveillance with clinical physical examinations and CA-125 at alternating visits with her oncologist and her surgeon.

Early detection and clinical awareness of the signs and symptoms of ovarian cancer will help to improve the relative survival of women with disease. It is important for physician assistants in the primary care setting to be aware of the subtle presentations and have an increased level of suspicion when a woman presents with these progressive, persistent, and frequent symptoms. It is recommended that those women with a family history of ovarian cancer seek genetic counseling and those with a BRCA gene mutation consider prophylactic surgery to reduce their ovarian cancer risk. Referral to a gynecologic oncologist early on will also help to optimize outcomes.

REFERENCES

1. National Cancer Institute. Surveillance, Epidemiology, and End Results Program. Available at: http://seer.cancer.gov/statfacts/html/ovary.html. Accessed January 31, 2016.
2. American Cancer Society. Survival rates for ovarian cancer, by stage. Available at: www.cancer.org/cancer/ovariancancer/detailedguide/ovarian-cancer-survival-rates. Accessed January 31, 2016.
3. NCCN Clinical Practice Guidelines in Oncology (NCCN Guidelines). Ovarian cancer including fallopian tube cancer and primary peritoneal cancer. Available at: www.nccn.org/professionals/physician_gls/pdf/ovarian.pdf. Accessed January 31, 2016.
4. American Cancer Society. What are the risk factors for ovarian cancer? Available at: www.cancer.org/cancer/ovariancancer/detailedguide/ovarian-cancer-risk-factors. Accessed January 31, 2016.
5. Finch A, Beiner M, Lubinski J, et al. Salpingo-oophorectomy and the risk of ovarian, fallopian tube, and peritoneal cancers in women with a BRCA1 or BRCA2 mutation. JAMA 2006;296(2):185–92.
6. American Congress of Obstetricians and Gynecologists. Women's health care physicians. Available at: www.acog.org/ResourcesAnd Publications/Committee Opinions/Committee on Gynecologic Practice/The Role of the Obstetrician Gynecologist in the Early Detection of Epithelial Ovarian Cancer.aspx. Accessed January 31, 2016.
7. Olson S, Mignone L, Nakraseive C, et al. Symptoms of ovarian cancer. Obstet Gynecol 2001;98(2):212–7.
8. Goff BA, Mandel L, Muntz HG, et al. Ovarian carcinoma diagnosis: results of a national ovarian cancer survey. Cancer 2000;89(10):2068–75.
9. Goff BA. Frequency of symptoms of ovarian cancer in women presenting to primary care clinics. JAMA 2004;291(22):2705.
10. Goff BA, Mandel LS, Drescher CW, et al. Development of an ovarian cancer symptom index. Cancer 2007;109(2):221–7.
11. American College of Obstetricians and Gynecologists Committee on Gynecologic Practice. Committee Opinion No. 477: the role of the obstetrician–gynecologist in the early detection of epithelial ovarian cancer. Obstet Gynecol 2011; 117(3):742–6.
12. Nurse Practitioners and Physician Assistants Advance Healthcare Networks. Early detection of ovarian cancer. Available at: http://nurse-practitioners-and-physician-assistants.advanceweb.com/Continuing-Education/CE-Articles/Early-Detection-of-Ovarian-Cancer.aspx. Accessed January 31, 2016.
13. Black A, Grubb RL III, Crawford ED. PLCO: a randomized controlled screening trial for prostate, lung, colorectal, and ovarian cancer. Prostate Cancer Screen 2009;361–72.
14. Clarke-Pearson DL. Screening for ovarian cancer. N Engl J Med 2009;361(2):170–7.

15. Walker RA. World Health Organization classification of tumours. Pathology and genetics of tumours of the breast and female genital organs. Histopathology 2005;46(2):229.
16. Kurman RJ, Shih I. The origin and pathogenesis of epithelial ovarian cancer: a proposed unifying theory. Am J Surg Pathol 2010;34(3):433–43.
17. Dietl J. Revisiting the pathogenesis of ovarian cancer: the central role of the fallopian tube. Arch Gynecol Obstet 2013;289(2):241–6.
18. Lawrie TA, Winter-Roach BA, Heus P, et al. Adjuvant (post-surgery) chemotherapy for early stage epithelial ovarian cancer. Cochrane Database Syst Rev 2015;(12):CD004706.
19. Society of Gynecologic Oncology. Genetic testing for ovarian cancer. 2014. Available at: www.sgo.org/clinical-practice/guidelines/genetic-testing-for-ovarian-cancer. Accessed January 31, 2016.
20. Ledermann J, Harter P, Gourley C, et al. Olaparib maintenance therapy in platinum-sensitive relapsed ovarian cancer. N Engl J Med 2012;366(15): 1382–92.
21. Chester C, Dorigo O, Berek JS, et al. Immunotherapeutic approaches to ovarian cancer treatment. J Immunother Cancer 2015;3(1):7.
22. Pardoll DM. The blockade of immune checkpoints in cancer immunotherapy. Nat Rev Cancer 2012;12(4):252–64.
23. Leach DR, Krummel MF, Allison JP. Enhancement of antitumor immunity by CTLA-4 blockade. Science 1996;271(5256):1734–6.
24. Cancer Research Institute. Ovarian cancer. 2015. Available at: www.cancerresearch.org/cancer-immunotherapy/impacting-all-cancers/ovarian-cancer. Accessed January 31, 2016.
25. Brentjens RJ, Davila ML, Riviere I, et al. CD19-targeted T cells rapidly induce molecular remissions in adults with chemotherapy-refractory acute lymphoblastic leukemia. Sci Transl Med 2013;5(177):177ra38.

Improving Access to Care: The Physician/Physician Assistant Team

Development of a Lymphoma-Specific Physician/Physician Assistant Team at a Comprehensive Cancer Center

Heather M. Hylton, MS, PA-C[a],*, Teresa G. Scardino, MPAS, PA-C[b]

KEYWORDS

- Patient-centered care • Team-based care • Care delivery model
- Team development • PA-lead initiatives • Walk-in clinic
- Optimizing scope of practice

KEY POINTS

- Although improvements in cancer care have been substantial over the past few decades, access to coordinated, high-quality cancer care remains a challenge for many patients due to several factors.
- An anticipated gap in supply and demand for cancer care services is anticipated in the coming decade, and Physician Assistants and Nurse Practitioners are poised to help meet the demand for these services.
- Given the increasing complexity of cancer care, there is growing interest in implementing a team-based approach to cancer care, and an optimally functioning team should have all members practicing to the fullest extent of their license, education, training, and competency.
- The authors propose a team-based approach to care as implemented in their Lymphoma Service, where PAs expand access for patients through multiple service-based initiatives.
- This model is adaptable and could be easily implemented in other areas of clinical practice.

INTRODUCTION

According to the American Cancer Society, 1,685,210 new cases of cancer are expected to be diagnosed in 2016, and 595,690 Americans will likely die from cancer this year.[1] Although these figures may seem staggering, significant

[a] Memorial Sloan Kettering Cancer Center (MSKCC), Department of Medicine, 1275 York Avenue, Box 124, New York, NY 10065, USA; [b] Memorial Sloan Kettering Cancer Center (MSKCC), Lymphoma Service, 205 East 64th Street, New York, NY 10065, USA
* Corresponding author.
E-mail address: hyltonh@mskcc.org

Physician Assist Clin 1 (2016) 489–497
http://dx.doi.org/10.1016/j.cpha.2016.03.004   physicianassistant.theclinics.com
2405-7991/16/$ – see front matter © 2016 Elsevier Inc. All rights reserved.

improvement in cancer survival has been made over the past few decades. In 1991, the number of cancer deaths peaked with 215 deaths from cancer occurring per 100,000 persons.[1] Decreases in smoking and improved ability to detect and treat cancers, however, have led to a substantial 23% decline in cancer deaths from 1991 to 2012, an overall decrease in cancer deaths of more than 1.7 million Americans.[1] As such, the 5-year survival rate for all cancers has improved from 49% for cancers diagnosed from 1975 to 1977 to 69% for cancers diagnosed from 2005 to 2011.[1]

Despite this progress, access to coordinated, high-quality care across the continuum of cancer care remains a challenge for many patients. According to the Institute of Medicine's 2013 report *Delivering High-Quality Cancer Care: Charting a New Course for a System in Crisis*, the following factors are likely to exacerbate current cancer care delivery issues[2]:

- An aging population
  - A 45% increase in the incidence of cancer by 2030 is anticipated
  - A 30% increase in survivors of cancer is anticipated from 2012 to 2022
- Workforce shortages
- Escalating cost of cancer care
  - The cost of cancer care in 2010 was $125 billion, up from $72 billion in 2004
  - In 2020, the cost of cancer care is projected to be approximately $173 billion
- Complexity associated with advances in understanding of cancer biology
- Limited availability and utilization of tools to improve quality of care

Furthermore, the uncertainty of the changing health care (and health care reform) landscape, reimbursement and productivity pressures, and importantly, provider burnout, have the potential to stress an already overwhelmed system and may pose additional barriers to patients' access to care.

SUPPLY AND DEMAND FOR CANCER CARE SERVICES

In 2007, the *Journal of Oncology Practice* published an analysis of the anticipated supply and demand for oncology services extending out to the year 2020. The study concluded the demand for oncology services is likely to significantly exceed the supply of services that could be provided, and a "multifaceted strategy" was recommended to address this shortfall.[3] In this landmark analysis, specific approaches to addressing this gap in supply and demand included increasing fellowship positions, postponing the retirement of oncologists currently in active clinical practice, eliminating inefficiencies in care delivery where possible, increasing primary care provider involvement in survivorship care, and increasing the utilization of Physician Assistants (PAs) and Nurse Practitioners (NPs) in care delivery.[3]

A follow-up analysis to the workforce study by Erikson and colleagues[3] was published in 2014 and confirmed the demand for oncology services is still expected to exceed the supply, and increasing productivity will be key. This study by Yang and colleagues[4] projected out to the year 2025, and while it was largely confirmatory of the earlier study by Erikson and colleagues,[3] the anticipated shortages may be somewhat delayed. Although the full impact of the Patient Protection and Affordable Care Act is yet unknown, this will likely also affect the demand for oncology services. Furthermore, the natural evolution in cancer treatment as a result of progress in research and how and where cancer care is delivered will also impact the demand for services.

BRIDGING THE GAP

With challenge comes opportunity, and PAs and NPs are poised to be a part of the solution to bridging the gap between supply and demand for oncology services. In the American Society of Clinical Oncology's Study of Collaborative Practice Arrangements, there were several key observations, which include[5]

- Patients were very satisfied with the care they received from a PA or NP and were aware when they were receiving care by a PA or NP.
- A 19% increase in productivity was seen in practices where PAs and NPs work with all the physicians (MDs) in the practice compared with a more exclusive model whereby PAs and NPs only work with a certain MD or MDs.
- A high level of satisfaction with their collaborative practice model was seen among both the MD and the PA/NP groups.

Although the findings from this study suggest satisfaction with collaborative practice arrangements among patients, MDs, and PAs and NPs, in the face of workforce shortages, there remains a significant challenge to recruitment and retention of PAs and NPs in oncology.[6] Ensuring proper mentorship of PAs and NPs is key; in a study by Ross and colleagues,[7] 91% of PAs indicated direct mentorship by their supervising MD was of primary importance to them.

In a recent quality of care–focused study by Glotzbecker and colleagues[8] comparing a traditional house staff–Attending MD team model to a PA–Attending MD team model, patient numbers and demographics on each team were comparable, and intensive care unit transfers and mortalities were similar across both groups. A statistically significant decrease in length of stay, readmission rates, and requested consults was seen on the PA-Attending MD team model, however, suggesting increased efficiency of the PA-Attending MD team model without compromising patient outcomes.[8]

THE ROLE OF PHYSICIAN ASSISTANTS IN ONCOLOGY

The very nature of the supervising MD–PA relationship lends itself to collaborative practice, and scope of practice for PAs is determined by state laws and regulations, facility policy, and delegation by the supervising MD. PAs practice in all subspecialty areas of adult medical and surgical oncology as well as radiation oncology and pediatric oncology. PAs deliver care in inpatient and outpatient settings, including the operating room, emergency centers, chemotherapy units, and hospice settings.[7] In addition to performing basic clinical functions, such as taking medical histories and performing physical examinations, PAs often function in expanded roles, including treatment planning, obtaining informed consent, performing or assisting with invasive procedures, prescribing chemotherapy and biologic therapy, and seeing new patient consultation visits.[7,9] As integral members of the oncology team, PAs provide services related to screening and diagnosis, supportive care during active treatment, survivorship care, and care at the end of life. PAs counsel patients on prevention, disease, and treatment; conduct goals of care and prognosis discussions; and may be active in clinical research activities/directly involved in Institutional Review Board–approved research.[7,9]

TEAM-BASED CARE IN ONCOLOGY

There is growing momentum for team-based care in oncology, and a highly performing team is essential for establishing and maintaining a coordinated, effective, and efficient health care delivery system that is patient-centric.[10] The 5 pillars of team-based health care include shared goals, clear roles, mutual trust, effective communication, and measurable processes and outcomes.[10] What distinguishes a group of providers caring for a patient from a team is the latter has a shared and valued goal toward which all individuals interact adaptively and dynamically and in an interdependent fashion to achieve this goal.[11]

To be effective, team-based care must be patient-centric and coordinated, with each member of the team having a clearly defined role. It is imperative for optimal functioning of the team that each member of the team is performing duties that are consistent with the fullest extent of the member's license (where applicable), education, training, and competency. Defining, as a team, each of the tasks that must be completed to provide optimal care to the patient is an exercise of great value. After defining these tasks, determination of the most appropriate member of the team to complete each identified task is paramount because this assures the patient's needs are being met by the most appropriate members of the team, provides role clarity and establishes accountability, and ensures each member of the team is performing at the functional level that is intended. This exercise also facilitates streamlining of workflows, which should reduce redundancy, improve efficiency, and avoid instances where tasks are not completed.

Team training has been shown to enhance team performance in health care delivery.[12–14] Each stakeholder in the patient's multidisciplinary care team, including MDs, PAs, NPs, nurses, pharmacists, social workers, rehabilitation specialists, support staff, and others, should be engaged and involved in team training interventions to set up such interventions for acceptance and success.[12] Tools such as the Agency for Healthcare Research and Quality's TeamSTEPPS (Strategies and Tools to Enhance Performance and Patient Safety) program are available to enhance teamwork skills to positively impact patient outcomes.[15,16] Key principles of TeamSTEPPs include team structure, communication, leadership, situation monitoring, and mutual support.[15] Further information about TeamSTEPPs can be found at http://www.ahrq.gov/professionals/education/curriculum-tools/teamstepps/index.html.

IMPLEMENTING A NEW CARE DELIVERY MODEL

To meet the needs of the authors' growing Lymphoma Service practice, expansion of capacity for patient visits was necessary. With the addition of a new Lymphoma Service Chief in early 2013 that had former experience with an MD/PA care model, the role of the lymphoma MD/PA care model began to fructify. Consequently, the Outpatient Lymphoma Service at Memorial Sloan Kettering Cancer Center (MSKCC) hired its first PA in June 2013, who came with 8 years of oncology experience, 4 of those years primarily with exposure to lymphoma patients in both the inpatient and the outpatient setting. Soon after, the second PA was hired and also came with 8 years of oncology experience.

Initially, there was some apprehension to deviate from a more MD-driven care model, although simultaneously, there was enthusiasm for a new care model, which held the potential to expand access to care. Currently, there are 5 outpatient PAs on the Lymphoma Service practicing full time; 4 are service-based and one has a primary focus in clinical research.

Before PAs were hired, the Outpatient Lymphoma Service at MSKCC mostly conformed to a MD-driven care model, working with fellows and office practice nurses. Fellow availability was variable, based on their rotation schedule. The staff attending MDs had less time to conduct much needed research in the field, an effort which is key to practice in an academic environment. In 2012, there were 12 practicing MDs. The MDs performed all new consultations and lymphoma-specific procedures, rounded on service inpatients, provided routine visits and mandatory investigational-specific follow-up as well as unplanned subacute visits. In addition, the MDs screened the patients for secondary effects of cancer treatments for many years after therapy.

With the integration of PAs into general Lymphoma Service operations, increased access for patients emerged through the creation of new clinics and extension of services that could be provided to patients.

PRACTICE MODELS

Currently, approximately 50% of the service-based PAs' clinical effort is directed toward supporting the practices of 2 designated MDs within the Lymphoma Service. The other 50% of the service-based PAs' clinical effort is directed toward supporting the needs of patients across the Lymphoma Service through various PA-driven clinics, which are described in this section. This general model of integration of PAs into the Lymphoma Service has evolved over time, both as understanding of PA practice has grown and as additional PAs have been added to the service.

Shared Clinic

The PAs each support an MD's clinic anywhere from 2 to 3 clinic days per week through conducting shared visits with the attending MD. Visit types seen during these clinics include new patient consultations, active and long-term follow-up visits, as well as treatment visits. The PA will typically initiate the patient encounter, gathering the medical history, performing a physical examination, and then presenting the patient to the attending. The patient's plan of care is discussed with the attending, who then sees the patient as well. There is also a certain level of care coordination outside of the nursing spectrum involving these patients, and this care facilitation and coordination are managed by the PAs. The shared clinic is an important aspect of the MD/PA care model to promote continuity of care for patients when their primary MD is absent from clinic due to inpatient rounding, travel, and the like.

Independent Clinic

Outside of shared clinic visits, the PAs see various types of patient encounters as independent visits, and the patient cohorts the PAs see in these visits are well-defined. The PAs currently conduct the following patient visits independently: lymphoma-specific procedures, survivorship visits, research-related visits, subacute/same-day add-ons, treatment encounters, as well as routine follow-up.

The first 2 PAs joined the Lymphoma Service mid-year in 2013. The third PA joined the Lymphoma Service mid-year in 2014, and 2 additional PAs, including the clinical research-focused PA, joined the service at the end of 2014. From 2013 to 2014, an approximately 5.3-fold increase in the volume of independent visits conducted by the PAs was seen; an additional approximately 1.8-fold increase in this volume from 2014 to 2015 was seen. In parallel, an incremental increase in new patient visits and follow-up visits for the service has been seen, suggesting expansion of the Outpatient Lymphoma PA Program has contributed to increasing patient access.

Lymphoma procedure clinic

In contrast to 2012 when the MDs were performing 100% of the Lymphoma Service procedures, now, other than the rare exception, almost all of the lymphoma-specific procedures are currently being performed by the PAs. These lymphoma-specific procedures specifically include lumbar punctures, Ommaya reservoir access, intrathecal chemotherapy administration, bone marrow aspiration and biopsies, and skin biopsies. These competencies are gained through intensive procedure training by a credentialed clinician. Procedures are scheduled separately from shared clinic time into a designated procedure clinic template. Each PA has a designated time slot for covering procedure clinic for ease of patient scheduling. From 2013 to 2015, more than a 5-fold increase in the number of procedures done by the PAs has been seen. Since integrating PAs into the Lymphoma Service in 2013, the overall volume of procedures has increased, while the number of procedures performed by MDs has decreased.

Survivorship clinic

As part of the longitudinal care provided to patients undergoing cancer treatment, it is necessary to monitor for the secondary long-term and late effects of cancer treatment sometimes for many years, depending on the treatment modality. At the authors' institution, they are committed to supporting patients physically, emotionally, and spiritually for as long as they need, and the Survivorship Clinic is embedded within the Lymphoma Service practice, which helps preserve continuity of care. The Lymphoma Survivorship Program was launched in 2014, designed for cancer survivors and their families, to monitor for the secondary effects of lymphoma treatment, which models the evidence-based American Society of Clinical Oncology's Cancer Treatment and Survivorship Care Plans. The patients are screened and monitored by the Lymphoma PAs autonomously after being remission for 2 years after treatment. They are typically seen every 6 months. Currently 2 of the 5 Lymphoma PAs accommodate survivorship visits in their schedule. With its implementation in 2014, the Lymphoma Survivorship Program at MSKCC has welcomed and successfully transitioned many patients into the program, which promotes a healthy and positive future after cancer treatment.

Walk-in clinic

In early 2015, the Outpatient Lymphoma Service piloted a walk-in clinic specifically for lymphoma patients. The Lymphoma Walk-In Clinic is likely one of the most notable initiatives to date due to its impact on the hospital system. Before opening the Lymphoma Walk-In Clinic, patient complaints were triaged between the clinical team and the Urgent Care Center (UCC). The UCC is MSKCC's "emergency room," whose care is specific to patients with cancer who are being seen and treated at the institution. It is not a public access emergency department. One of the goals of instituting the Walk-In Clinic was to increase access for patients who needed to be seen on the same day but who did not necessarily require treatment in an acute care setting.

In 2014, a multidisciplinary team of MDs, PAs, nurses, and administration came together to develop a workflow designed to provide comprehensive subacute care to patients in the outpatient lymphoma setting in an attempt reduce UCC admissions. In this workflow, patient complaints are evaluated by the Office Practice Nurse, along with the PA if necessary, to determine if the patient meets the criteria to be seen in the Lymphoma Walk-In Clinic. By executing this multidisciplinary workflow, lymphoma patients are now able to receive same-day care for subacute needs from a familiar clinical team in an outpatient setting. The Lymphoma Walk-In Clinic has impacted the institution by decreasing urgent care visits and subsequent hospital admissions as well as providing increased access to treatment of subacute medical conditions for lymphoma patients, and patient satisfaction with the Walk-In Clinic has been high.

In addition, the Lymphoma Walk-In Clinic has, at times, also served as a bridge to acute care in the cases where this level of care was ultimately needed. For example, a patient presented to the Walk-In Clinic for evaluation, and workup led to a UCC admission for suspected sepsis. Although a UCC admission was still necessary in this case, the patient workup was initiated in the Walk-In Clinic and the patient was able to begin antibiotics promptly in the outpatient setting, which streamlined care on arrival to the UCC.

Furthermore, this has resulted in an overall decrease in wait times for patients who are seeking care for lymphoma- or lymphoma treatment-related issues. Patients have expressed appreciation for the convenience and accessibility of medical care received in the Lymphoma Walk-In Clinic. Last, this model received recognition from the authors' institution's Division of Quality and Safety at the 2015 Quality and Performance Improvement event.

SUMMARY/DISCUSSION

As additional PAs have been integrated into the ambulatory Lymphoma Service practice at the authors' institution, expansion of services offered to patients has been achievable. In addition, they have thoughtfully composed the team in each aspect of care delivery, leveraging diverse skill sets and experiential backgrounds for the benefit of the patients, the service, and the institution, and aligning interests and opportunities for PA leadership in service initiatives.

Multiple factors have contributed to the success of this model. The first factor is the willingness to adapt the model in order to fully use the appropriated resources. The model continues to evolve as the authors work to establish best practices for patient care within the changing health care landscape. Another point of interest of this model is that it has shown itself to be a productive model. Although many practices are looking to identify appropriate productivity benchmarks for PAs and NPs, there is no established "gold standard" for productivity to date. PAs and NPs often have a considerable role in coordination of care, and generally these activities, while adding value, are difficult to measure, although provision of these services is necessary to provide the highest quality care for the patient. PAs and NPs must become adept at understanding the business aspects of medicine, including the concepts of productivity and value, and understand what they bring to the table above and beyond productivity measurements.[17]

Productivity, in general, is further enhanced through ensuring appropriate clinic support and infrastructure. This productivity relates, in part, back to the key components of highly functional teams. The model is also notable in that approximately 50% of each service-based PA's time and effort is dedicated to clinical activities that benefit the Lymphoma Service patients as a whole (ie, Walk-In Clinic, procedure clinics, and survivorship clinics), while the other 50% of each service-based PA's time is allocated to working in specific MD practices; this relates back to the findings of increased productivity seen in practices where PAs and NPs worked with all the MDs in the practice.[5] Also notable is that the patient cohorts the PAs see in independent visits are clearly defined. Where applicable, the PA/MD team may wish to establish guidelines in the practice regarding the visit frequency to the PA and the MD. For example, the patient may see the MD every third or fourth visit and see the PA at all other visits.

Last, a key to the success of this model has been the continued work to optimize the PAs' scope of practice. Ideally, the scope of practice for a PA is determined at the practice level, and facility policy should align with state laws and regulations governing PA practice. Clinical privileges should be appropriate for the care to be delivered, and performance evaluation through such processes as focused professional practice evaluation and ongoing professional practice evaluation should be used to document competency.

This article provides one example of an MD/PA care delivery model in a comprehensive cancer center. Although the current model continues to evolve alongside the expansion of resources, the outlined process has been deemed successful as judged by the depicted benchmarks. Explicitly, there has been an increase in service productivity, broadening of patient care services provided, enhanced access to care, improved continuity of care, and a decreased impact on the system through decanting UCC referrals where appropriate.

REFERENCES

1. American Cancer Society. Cancer facts & figures 2016. Atlanta (GA): American Cancer Society; 2016.
2. Institute of Medicine. Delivering high-quality cancer care: charting a new course for a system in crisis. Washington, DC: National Academies Press; 2013.
3. Erikson C, Salsberg E, Forte G, et al. Future supply and demand for oncologists. J Oncol Pract 2007;3(2):79–86.
4. Yang W, Williams JH, Hogan PF, et al. Projected supply of and demand for oncologists and radiation oncologists through 2025: an aging, better-insured population will result in shortage. J Oncol Pract 2014;10(1): 39–45.
5. Towle EL, Barr TH, Hanley A, et al. Results of the ASCO study of collaborative practice arrangements. J Oncol Pract 2011;7(5):278–82.
6. Coniglio D, Pickard T, Wei S. Commentary: physician assistant perspective on the results of the ASCO study of collaborative practice arrangements. J Oncol Pract 2011;7(5):283–4.
7. Ross AC, Polansky MN, Parker PA, et al. Understanding the role of physician assistants in oncology. J Oncol Pract 2010;6(1):26–30.
8. Glotzbecker BE, Yolin-Raley DS, DeAngelo DJ, et al. Impact of physician assistants on the outcomes of patients with acute myelogenous leukemia receiving chemotherapy in an academic medical center. J Oncol Pract 2013; 9(5):e228–33.
9. Hylton HM. Clinical partnership: the role of physician assistants in oncology practice. ASCO Daily News 2011;21B.
10. Mitchell P, Wynia M, Golden R, et al. Core principles & values of effective team-based health care. Washington, DC: Institute of Medicine; 2012.
11. Taplin SH, Weaver S, Chollette V, et al. Teams and teamwork during a cancer diagnosis: interdependency within and between teams. J Oncol Pract 2015; 11(3):231–8.
12. Bunnell CA, Gross AH, Weingart SN, et al. High performance teamwork training and systems redesign in outpatient oncology. BMJ Qual Saf 2013; 22:405–13.
13. Salas E, Rosen MA. Building high reliability teams: progress and some reflections on teamwork training. BMJ Qual Saf 2013;22:369–73.
14. Jones KJ, Skinner AM, High R, et al. A theory-driven, longitudinal evaluation of the impact of team training on safety culture in 24 hospitals. BMJ Qual Saf 2013;22:394–404.
15. Agency for Healthcare Research and Quality. TeamSTEPPS 2.0 Pocket Guide: team strategies & tools to enhance performance and patient safety. Washington, DC: Agency for Healthcare Research and Quality; 2013.

16. Weaver SJ, Dy SM, Rosen MA. Team-training in healthcare: a narrative synthesis of the literature. BMJ Qual Saf 2014;0:1–14.
17. Pickard T. Calculating your worth: understanding productivity and value. J Adv Pract Oncol 2014;5:128–33.

SUGGESTED READINGS

American Society of Clinical Oncology. The state of cancer care in America. Alexandria (Virginia): American Society of Clinical Oncology; 2016. Available at: http://read.uberflip.com/i/653313-socca-2016-flipbook.
Taplin SH, Weaver S, Salas E, et al. Reviewing cancer care team effectiveness. J Oncol Pract 2015;11(3):239–46.

Surgical Options for Post-Mastectomy Breast Reconstruction

Brittney O'Grady, MMS, PA-C

KEYWORDS

- Breast cancer • Autologous • Reconstruction • Prosthesis

KEY POINTS

- The aim of the present article is to provide a brief review of prosthesis-based and autologous-based breast reconstruction.
- The article focuses on the timeline behind reconstruction, the effect of radiation, and manner in which the appropriate surgical method is based on patient selection, sound clinical judgment, and surgical technique.
- Regarding autologous reconstruction, the review provides a brief summary behind the factors optimizing success as well as the role of the physician assistant in flap-based reconstruction.

Typically, women think about their breasts at least once a day: the attempt to secure them, a need to lift them, the pressure to artificially pump them to super-human proportions. It is a love-hate relationship that flowers into existence with adolescent breast buds and ultimately transforms into something with both social and scientific significance. Breasts are more than just organs; they are laden with hugely powerful and provocative meanings to men and women alike. Therefore, what happens when cancer takes them?

For most women, breast cancer is a sudden and unpredicted diagnosis found only during a routine breast examination. This diagnosis is a time of numbing anxiety, riddled with fear of the unknown and constant thoughts of worst-case scenarios. However, a cadre of niche patients can plan ahead. Patients who inherit the deleterious BRCA mutation, a gene known to cause breast cancer, will often elect to have bilateral mastectomies based on their high-risk status.[1] These patients are often younger[2] and do not have active cancer and therefore do not require radiation or chemotherapy.

Disclosure: None.
MD Anderson Cancer Center, Department of Plastic Surgery, 1400 Pressler St, Houston TX 77030, USA
E-mail address: baogrady@mdanderson.org

Physician Assist Clin 1 (2016) 499–509
http://dx.doi.org/10.1016/j.cpha.2016.03.008
2405-7991/16/$ – see front matter Published by Elsevier Inc.

In terms of public awareness, Angelina Jolie has become to BRCA-associated breast cancer roughly what Lance Armstrong was to testicular cancer in the 1990s. Her diagnosis has caused an influx of women to be tested for the gene and even request bilateral mastectomies. This dramatic increase in awareness has been dubbed "The Jolie Effect".[3] In 2013, she underwent bilateral prophylactic mastectomies, and her reconstruction was done in a remarkable fashion, a one-step procedure. She underwent a nipple-sparing mastectomy, which directly proceeded to implant. However, her case is not the "norm." Jolie had no comorbidities and no active cancer. She reported finishing her entire breast reconstruction in a remarkable timeframe, 9 weeks. Most patients' final reconstruction takes anywhere from 9 months to a year and even longer in some cases.[4]

It is imperative women know their options for breast reconstruction and what, in fact, is a reasonable timetable. Breast reconstruction is not a one-size-fits-all surgery or algorithm and, regardless of BRCA status, is often a long and arduous journey. Reconstruction is based on the individual and their personal journey toward self-reinvention.

BREAST CANCER OVERVIEW

Breast cancer is the leading cause of cancer death among women worldwide, and hereditary cancers (such as BRCA1 and BRCA2) account for 5% to 10% of all breast cancer.[5,6] The treatment options for patients with breast cancer are complex and varied. Options range from surveillance and chemoprevention to adjuvant and neoadjuvant cytotoxic cocktails, targeted immunotherapy, radiation, and surgery. A multimodal management plan is often implemented with good effect. Advances in screening, prevention, treatment, and supportive care continue to improve cure rates, increase the number of breast cancer survivors, and improve quality of life. A detailed review of the pathophysiology and management of breast cancer is beyond the scope of this review; however, the interested reader is directed toward the National Comprehensive Cancer Network's Clinical Practice Guidelines in Oncology for Breast Cancer. These evidence-based guidelines include up-to-date, best practice standards for the clinical management of patients with carcinoma in situ, invasive breast cancer, Paget disease, Phyllodes tumor, inflammatory breast cancer, or breast cancer during pregnancy.[7]

STAGING SYSTEM

A detailed history and physical examination remain the foundation of breast cancer staging, the primary TNM. The TNM system is the most extended scheme of stage grouping in cancer. Stage grouping summarizes the anatomic extension of a cancer at the moment of diagnosis and is based on 3 components: the T (primary tumor growth), the N (local lymph node involvement), and the M (distant metastasis). Stage grouping classifies cancers into stages: stage I (small or superficial localized cancer), stage II (large or deep localized cancer), stage III (regionally spread cancer), and stage IV (cancer with distant metastasis).[8,9] These stages are determined based on physical examination, mammogram, ultrasound, MRIs, blood work, and tissue abnormality.

After the diagnosis and staging, a multidisciplinary approach to surgical treatment (radical, modified, or segmental mastectomies) and therapeutic treatment (breast irradiation techniques and systemic cytotoxic and hormonal therapy) is determined.[10,11] This article focuses on breast reconstruction in the form of implants and autologous tissue.

BREAST RECONSTRUCTION AFTER MASTECTOMY
Skin-Sparing and Nipple-Sparing Mastectomy

A mastectomy is the surgical procedure done to remove the breast tissue. In the past, a radical mastectomy (removal of the breast tissue, nipple, lymph nodes, and the chest wall muscles) was the standard of care for breast cancer. However, this is rarely the case in the twenty-first century, except in the setting of aggressive disease. Today, the skin (skin-sparing mastectomy) and nipple (nipple-sparing mastectomy) are often spared. These surgical approaches compared with radical mastectomies have been found to have equivalent long-term outcomes with equivalent survival and recurrence rates.[12,13]

However, in regards to a nipple-sparing approach, the debate over the appropriate surgical indications and patient selection continues to evolve. Currently, many surgeons offer nipple-sparing mastectomy only to patients who have a peripheral tumor less than 3 cm in diameter with no nodal disease, and some studies recommend that nipple-sparing mastectomy be performed only in patients who have tumors no closer than 5 cm to the nipple-areola complex.[14] Selection criteria must also include the anatomy of the breast itself, since patients with larger or more ptotic-shaped breasts are more likely to have nipple or flap necrosis.[15] The popularity of these techniques has a direct correlation with patient expectations, and optimum cosmetic outcomes in breast reconstruction also increased.[16–18]

Radiation

The need for radiation is determined on the basis of several variables and factors and is continuously evolving. The treatment plan is often determined once pathology results are available. The threshold for radiation varies from institution to institution. The need for radiation has a tremendous impact on the reconstructive algorithm and can drastically affect the final cosmetic result. Following radiation, the soft tissue undergoes dramatic changes secondary to damage to the microcirculation leading to less well-perfused tissue. The skin often becomes more fibrotic and consequently more prone to complications, such as infection, delayed wound healing, implant extrusion, and capsular contracture.[19] For these reasons, most reconstructive surgeons recommend using autologous tissue in the setting of prior radiation.[20]

Expander-Implant-Based Reconstruction

Several innovations in reconstruction are designed to optimize breast skin survival. The most common means of breast reconstruction following a mastectomy is using a tissue expander and implant approach. After a skin-sparing or nipple-sparing mastectomy, the perfusion to the remaining breast skin is compromised due to the removal of the breast tissue and perforators, which directly supply the skin. For this reason, a tissue expander is often placed at the time of the mastectomy in order to preserve the remaining breast skin. The design of the expander is similar to that of a depleted implant and aids in preserving the skin envelope and minimizing skin flap necrosis (**Fig. 1**). The tissue expander is typically placed in the subpectoral location in order to provide total soft tissue coverage for protection of the expander and minimize any pressure directly against the skin.[21]

In the setting that the pectoralis major muscle is inadequate to provide complete coverage of the expander, the use of acellular dermal matrix (ADM) is now becoming the standard of care. The ADM can be derived from several different sources including fetal bovine or porcine dermis as well as human cadavers.[22–24] The ADM is inset as an inferior sling along the inferior pole of the breast. The concept of using these products

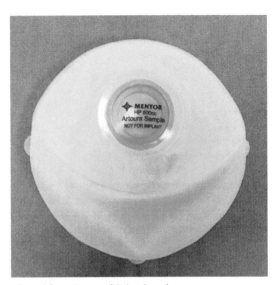

Fig. 1. Tissue expander with an integral injection dome.

is to provide support and total coverage of the expander to minimize any pressure on the mastectomy skin flaps that can precipitate skin necrosis and compromise the final esthetic result of the reconstruction.[25–27] An example of postoperative widespread mastectomy skin flap necrosis is illustrated in **Fig. 2**.

The expander is then inflated to the size the patient desires or to the limits of skin tolerance (**Fig. 3**). Once the expansion process is completed, the patient needs to undergo a second procedure in order to exchange the expander for a permanent

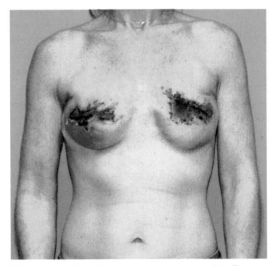

Fig. 2. A 44-year-old woman with widespread mastectomy skin flap necrosis and cellulitis. She is postoperative 2 weeks from bilateral mastectomies with immediate reconstruction using the placement of tissue expanders, Mentor Artoura 375 cc capacity with the intraoperative fill of 100 cc of saline, and placement of bioprosthetic mesh. (*Courtesy of* Jesse C. Selber, MD, MPH, FACS.)

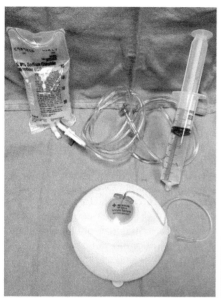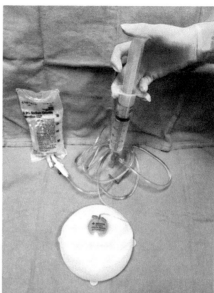

Fig. 3. The tissue expander is inserted intraoperatively (underfilled), and over time sterile saline fluid is added by inserting a small needle through the skin and into the tissue expander port. As the tissue expander fills, the skin will stretch and create the new breast pocket.

implant. Implants are available in several different sizes and vary in volume, width, and projection. The implants range from round to anatomic and from saline to silicone.[28,29] The anatomic shape is meant to mimic the shape of a native breast, and they are gaining popularity (**Fig. 4**). The entire process is variable but can be lengthy depending on

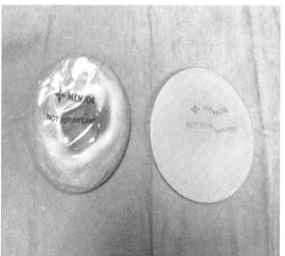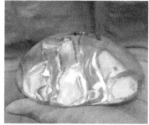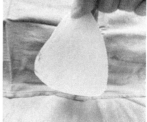

Fig. 4. Example of silicone implants (*left*). The top right is a smooth, round implant with a uniform round profile. The bottom right is a textured, anatomic implant with a teardrop profile.

the need for adjuvant chemotherapy and radiation. Both of these adjuvant therapies can delay definitive reconstruction anywhere from 6 months to a year.[30–32]

Autologous-Based Reconstruction

In the setting of prior radiation, autologous tissue is recommended to minimize the risks of complications. Using autologous tissue to reconstruct the breast uses tissue from another part of the body to re-create an esthetic breast mound and is referred to as a flap. There are several different sites where tissue can be used in order to rebuild a breast. The most common donor sites are discussed in subsequent sections: transverse rectus abdominus myocutaneous (TRAM) flap/deep inferior epigastric perforator (DIEP) flap, latissimus dorsi myocutaneous flap. The decision to proceed with a specific flap technique is based on many different factors, including available tissue and desired breast size, recovery time and duration of surgery, other medial comorbidities and prior surgeries, patient preference, and surgeon experience.

Transverse Rectus Abdominus Myocutaneous Flap/Deep Inferior Epigastric Perforator

The abdomen represents the most common and most popular donor site.[33,34] The consistency of the fat and skin of the abdomen most closely approximates that of breast tissue, and most patients have enough laxity in the abdomen to harvest sufficient tissue to rebuild a breast.[35] An example of a postoperative outcome following unilateral breast reconstruction using a DIEP flap is illustrated in **Fig. 5**.

The tissue from the abdomen can be harvested with or without muscle and can be transferred as a pedicle flap or a free flap. A free abdominal flap is separated from its native blood supply and reconnected to new blood vessels in the chest, and a pedicled flap maintains its blood from the abdomen and is tunneled into the chest and then shaped into the breast shape. When no muscle is harvested with the flap, the

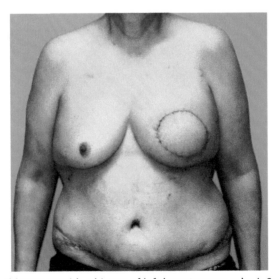

Fig. 5. A 55-year-old woman with a history of left breast cancer, who is 2 weeks status post single perforator DIEP to the left breast. She will undergo possible revisions to the free flap and a contralateral breast augmentation for symmetry in 3 months. (*Courtesy of* Jesse C. Selber, MD, MPH, FACS.)

flap is considered a DIEP flap; however, variable amounts of muscle may need to be harvested resulting in a muscle-sparing TRAM flap. A free flap divides the blood vessels supplying the tissue and requires the blood vessels to be reconnected, most commonly to the internal mammary vessels to maintain perfusion of the tissue.[36] The thoracodorsal vessels historically were the recipient vessels of choice, but the internal mammary vessels are now considered the more ideal vessels.[37] The internal mammary vessels allow medial positioning of the flap, due to their anatomic location on the chest wall, and also preserve the latissimus dorsi flap in the setting of a flap loss.

In general, a free flap is more challenging and is a longer operation; however, they are the standard of care at most high-volume institutions, although the pedicle TRAM is the most commonly performed operation for autologous tissue breast reconstruction.[38]

Closure of the donor site is as critical as shaping and reconstruction of an esthetic breast mound and oftentimes occurs simultaneously with the microsurgical portion of the operation. A 2-team approach is often helpful to limit the operative time, and physician assistants play a critical role in improving the efficiency in the operating room. Physician assistants can function as a first assist and also have the surgical skills to work autonomously, such as closing the abdominal donor site while the surgeon is working on the breast. The fascia is closed with a permanent suture and occasionally may require reinforcement with mesh in order to minimize the risks of developing a hernia following flap harvest. Mesh is often warranted in the setting of bilateral breast reconstruction, when both the lateral and the medial rows are harvested, or when a full muscle TRAM and not a DIEP is performed.[39,40]

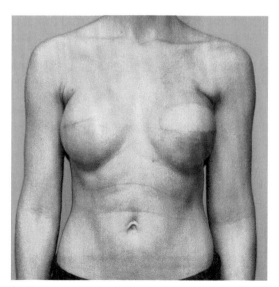

Fig. 6. A 32-year-old (body mass index, 19.5) woman postoperative 3 weeks status post placement of bilateral implants, Mentor 350 cc smooth round high profile silicone implants. She has a history of left breast cancer, T1N3c, chemotherapy, bilateral mastectomies, and radiation therapy to the left chest wall. Reconstruction was completed in 2 stages, bilateral tissue expanders with a left pedicled myocutaneous latissimus dorsi flap and exchange of tissue expanders for implants. She will undergo bilateral 3D nipple areolar micropigmentation in 3 months. (*Courtesy of* Jesse C. Selber, MD, MPH, FACS.)

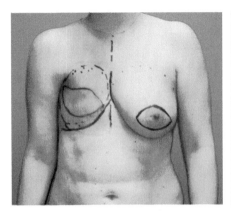
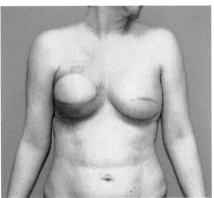

Fig. 7. A 33-year-old woman who underwent a right-sided mastectomy, no reconstruction and radiation therapy. Nine months after radiation, she underwent delayed reconstruction in the form of a left latissimus dorsi myocutaneous flap, right breast mastectomy, and bilateral placement of tissue expanders. (*Left*) Preoperative frontal view with surgical markings. (*Right*) Postoperative 2 months and undergoing tissue expansions. (*Courtesy of* Jesse C. Selber, MD, MPH, FACS.)

Pedicled Latissimus Dorsi Myocutaneous Flap

For patients that do not have adequate soft tissue in the abdomen or the gluteal region, a pedicled latissimus dorsi flap is the recommended option to supplement the reconstruction (**Fig. 6**). However, because the latissimus dorsi often does not have the same bulk and adiposity as the abdomen, this form of reconstruction typically requires placement of an implant as well.[41]

This surgery is considerably shorter than a free TRAM/DIEP and takes about 5 hours. During surgery, the latissimus dorsi muscle is released from its attachments to the iliac crest, its posterior attachments, and subsequently, the superior attachments, separating the latissimus dorsi flap away from the trapezius.[42] An elevated tunnel between the breast and the latissimus dorsi donor site is used to pass the flap into the breast, without compressing the pedicle. In the setting of radiation, this flap provides healthy vascularized soft tissue coverage for the prosthesis and minimizes the chance of developing complications (**Fig. 7**). The physician assistant will close the donor site in this operation as well.

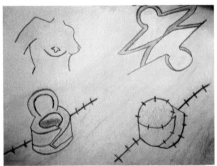
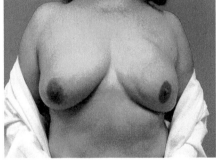

Fig. 8. Modified C-V flap (*left*). A 45-year-old patient status post TRAM flap to the left breast with nipple reconstruction using the C-V flap technique and nipple areolar micropigmentation (*right*). (*Courtesy of* Jesse C. Selber, MD, MPH, FACS.)

Nipple Reconstruction

Nipple-areola reconstruction completes the breast reconstruction process, significantly enhances esthetic outcomes and body image and restores the patient's feeling of wholeness.[43,44] Various techniques can be used, including composite nipple grafts, local flap, flaps with autologous graft augmentation, flaps with alloplastic augmentation, and flaps with allograft augmentation and 3-dimensional (3D) nipple areolar micropigmentation.[45] A local nipple flap (**Fig. 8**) with tattooing of the areola is currently the most singular methods.[46] However, the type of surgical technique performed will depend on the skin integrity as well as the surgeon and patient preference.

SUMMARY

In the end, it is about getting back what cancer took. Breast reconstruction is at the heart of plastic surgery. An implant-based approach and an autologous approach both provide excellent results, and techniques continue to evolve. Reconstructive limits are constantly being pushed and boundaries are being tested, in hopes of helping patients feel whole again.

REFERENCES

1. Angelos P, Bedrosian I, Euhus DM, et al. Contralateral prophylactic mastectomy: challenging considerations for the surgeon. Ann Surg Oncol 2015 Oct;22(10): 3208–12.

2. Stucky CC, Gray RJ, Wasif N, et al. Increase in contralateral prophylactic mastectomy: echoes of a bygone era? Surgical trends for unilateral breast cancer. Ann Surg Oncol 2010;17(Suppl 3):330–7.

3. Borzekowski DL, Guan Y, Smith KC, et al. The Angelina effect: immediate reach, grasp, and impact going public. Genet Med 2014;16:516–21.

4. MD Anderson Cancer Center. Reshaping you. Houston (TX): MD Anderson Cancer Center; 2010.

5. Torre LA, Bray F, Siegel RL, et al. Global cancer statistics, 2012. CA Cancer J Clin 2015;65(2):87–108.

6. Cordeiro PG. Breast reconstruction after surgery for breast cancer. N Engl J Med 2008;359(15):1590–601.

7. Gradishar WJ, Anderson BO, Balassanian R. Breast cancer, version 1.2016. J Natl Compr Canc Netw 2015;13:1475–85.

8. Sobin LH, Gospodarowicz MK, Wittekind C. TNM classification of malignant tumors. 7. Oxford (United Kingdom): Wiley-Blackwell; 2010.

9. Ramos M, Franch P, Zaforteza M, et al. Completeness of T, N, M and stage grouping for all cancers in the Mallorca cancer registry. BMC Cancer 2015; 15:847.

10. Cody HS. Current surgical management of breast cancer. Curr Opin Obstet Gynecol 2002;14(1):45–52.

11. Sakorafas GH. Breast cancer surgery–historical evolution, current status and future perspectives. Acta Oncol 2001;40:186–284.

12. Colwell AS, Tessler O, Lin AM, et al. Breast reconstruction following nipple-sparing mastectomy: predictors of complications, reconstruction outcomes, and 5-year trends. Plast Reconstr Surg 2014;133(3):496–506.

13. Wang F, Peled AW, Garwood E, et al. Total skin-sparing mastectomy and immediate breast reconstruction: an evolution of technique and assessment of outcomes. Ann Surg Oncol 2014;21(10):3223–30.

14. Gould DJ, Hunt KK, Liu J, et al. Impact of surgical techniques, biomaterials, and patient variables on rate of nipple necrosis after nipple-sparing mastectomy. Plast Reconstr Surg 2013;132:330e–8e.

15. Spear SL, Hannan CM, Willey SC, et al. Nipple-sparing mastectomy. Plast Reconstr Surg 2009;123:1665–73.

16. Salgarello M, Farallo E. Immediate breast reconstruction with definitive anatomical implants after skin-sparing mastectomy. Br J Plast Surg 2005;58:216–22.

17. Edlich RF, Winters KL, Faulkner BC, et al. Advances in breast reconstruction after mastectomy. J Long Term Eff Med Implants 2005;15(2):197–207.

18. Endara M, Chen D, Verma K, et al. Breast reconstruction following nipple-sparing mastectomy: a systematic review of the literature with pooled analysis. Plast Reconstr Surg 2013;132(5):1043–54.

19. Hvilsom GB, Holmich LR, Steding-Jessen M, et al. Delayed breast implant reconstruction: is radiation therapy associated with capsular contracture or reoperations? Ann Plast Surg 2012;68:246–52.

20. Anker CJ, Hymas RV, Ahluwalia R, et al. The effect of radiation on complication rates and patient satisfaction in breast reconstruction using temporary tissue expanders and permanent implants. Breast J 2015;21(3):233–40.

21. Radovan C. Breast reconstruction after mastectomy using the temporary expander. Plast Reconstr Surg 1982;69(2):195–208.

22. Spear SL, Sher SR, Al-Attar A. Focus on technique: supporting the soft-tissue envelope in breast reconstruction. Plast Reconstr Surg 2012;130(5 Suppl 2):89S–94S.

23. Ibrahim AM, Koolen PG, Ganor O, et al. Does acellular dermal matrix really improve aesthetic outcome in tissue expander/implant-based breast reconstruction? Aesthetic Plast Surg 2015;39(3):359–68.

24. Pannucci CJ, Antony AK, Wilkins EG. The impact of acellular dermal matrix on tissue expander/implant loss in breast reconstruction: an analysis of the tracking outcomes and operations in plastic surgery database. Plast Reconstr Surg 2013;132(1):1–10.

25. Selber JC, Wren JH, Garvey PB, et al. Critical evaluation of risk factors and early complications in 564 consecutive two-stage implant-based breast reconstructions using acellular dermal matrix at a single center. Plast Reconstr Surg 2015;136(1):10–20.

26. Crosby MA, Dong W, Feng L, et al. Effect of intraoperative saline fill volume on perioperative outcomes in tissue expander breast reconstruction. Plast Reconstr Surg 2011;127(3):1065–72.

27. Phillips BT, Lanier ST, Conkling N, et al. Intraoperative perfusion techniques can accurately predict mastectomy skin flap necrosis in breast reconstruction: results of a prospective trial. Plast Reconstr Surg 2012;129(5):778e–88e.

28. Nahabedian MY. Shaped versus round implants for breast reconstruction: indications and outcomes. Plast Reconstr Surg Glob Open 2014;2(3):e116.

29. Hedén P, Montemurro P, Adams WP Jr, et al. Anatomical and round breast implants: how to select and indications for use. Plast Reconstr Surg 2015;136(2):263–72.

30. Maxwell GP, Gabriel A. The evolution of breast implants. Plast Reconstr Surg 2014;134(Suppl 1):12S–7S.

31. Alderman A, Gutowski K, Ahuja A, et al, Postmastectomy Expander Implant Breast Reconstruction Guideline Work Group. ASPS Clinical Practice Guideline summary on breast reconstruction with expanders and implants. Plast Reconstr Surg 2014;134(4):648e–55e.

32. Peled AW, Foster RD, Esserman LJ, et al. Increasing the time to expander-implant exchange after postmastectomy radiation therapy reduces expander-implant failure. Plast Reconstr Surg 2012;130(3):503–9.

33. Massey MF, Spiegel AJ, Levine JL, et al, Group for the Advancement of Breast Reconstruction. Perforator flaps: recent experience, current trends, and future directions based on 3974 microsurgical breast reconstructions. Plast Reconstr Surg 2009 Sep;124(3):737–51.

34. Chang DW, Barnea Y, Robb GL. Effects of an autologous flap combined with an implant for breast reconstruction: an evaluation of 1000 consecutive reconstructions of previously irradiated breasts. Plast Reconstr Surg 2008;122:356–62.

35. Kronowitz SJ. Current status of autologous tissue-based breast reconstruction in patients receiving postmastectomy radiation therapy. Plast Reconstr Surg 2012; 130:282–92.

36. Chang EI, Chang EI, Soto-Miranda MA, et al. Demystifying the use of internal mammary vessels as recipient vessels in free flap breast reconstruction. Plast Reconstr Surg 2013;132(4):763–8.

37. Saint-Cyr M, Youssef A, Bae HW, et al. Changing trends in recipient vessel selection for microvascular autologous breast reconstruction: an analysis of 1483 consecutive cases. Plast Reconstr Surg 2007;119(7):1993–2000.

38. Nelson JA, Guo Y, Sonnad SS, et al. A comparison between DIEP and muscle-sparing free TRAM flaps in breast reconstruction: a single surgeon's recent experience. Plast Reconstr Surg 2010;126(5):1428–35.

39. Selber JC, Serletti JM. The deep inferior epigastric perforator flap: myth and reality. Plast Reconstr Surg 2010;125(1):50–8.

40. Garvey PB, Salavati S, Feng L, et al. Abdominal donor-site outcomes for medial versus lateral deep inferior epigastric artery branch perforator harvest. Plast Reconstr Surg 2011;127(6):2198–205.

41. Kronowitz SJ, Robb GL, Youssef A, et al. Optimizing autologous breast reconstruction in thin patients. Plast Reconstr Surg 2003;112(7):1768–78.

42. Gray H, Goss CM. Anatomy of the human body. Philadelphia: Lea & Febiger; 1973.

43. Ainslie NB, Ojeda-Fournier H. Creating a realistic breast: the nipple-areola reconstruction. Plast Surg Nurs 1996;16(3):156–61.

44. El-Ali K, Dalal M, Kat CC. Modified C-V flap for nipple reconstruction: our results in 50 patients. J Plast Reconstr Aesthet Surg 2009;62(8):991–6.

45. Nimboriboonporn A, Chuthapisith S. Nipple-areola complex reconstruction. Gland Surg 2014;3(1):35–42.

46. Boccola MA, Savage J, Rozen WM, et al. Surgical correction and reconstruction of the nipple-areola complex: current review of techniques. J Reconstr Microsurg 2010;26(9):589–600.

Ethical Considerations in Oncology

Sharyn L. Kurtz, PA-C, MPAS, MA

KEYWORDS

- Ethics/bioethics • Values • Treatment refusal • Moral distress
- Surrogate decision making • Nonbeneficial therapy • Parental permission/assent

KEY POINTS

- The physician assistant (PA) has a unique role within the interdisciplinary care team and is required to provide comprehensive care for the oncology patient.
- The quantity of time a PA spends providing clinical care for an oncology patient allows the PA access to particular knowledge of the patient's medical condition and social/religious/cultural values.
- Because of the complex nature of cancer care and the diverse needs of oncology patients, PAs often encounter ethical dilemmas while providing care for cancer patients.
- PAs benefit from knowledge about common ethical dilemmas encountered in the care of oncology patients and about approaches pertaining to ethical deliberation.

INTRODUCTION

The care needs of oncology patients are complex and require clinicians to extend beyond routine clinical decision making. Certain clinical situations may leave a PA asking, "What is the right thing to do?" Such inquiries involve examining the ethical considerations of cancer care. Ethical considerations are separate from what is permitted by law and instead focus on what is morally right or wrong. The term, *bioethics*, can be defined as the best moral course of action in a health care situation.[1] In other words, "What should I do for my patient?"

This article focuses on 3 patient cases, with the goal of highlighting common ethical considerations in the care of cancer patients. Each case is authentic in nature; however, the cases have been deidentified to maintain the privacy of those involved. The patient cases also provide examples for ethical deliberation as a means for mediating ethical conflicts. The PA role in bioethics also is discussed.

Disclosure Statement: The author has no disclosures to report.
Memorial Sloan Kettering Cancer Center, Department of Medicine, Lymphoma Service, 1275 York Avenue, New York, NY 10065, USA
E-mail address: kurtzs@mskcc.org

Physician Assist Clin 1 (2016) 511–522
http://dx.doi.org/10.1016/j.cpha.2016.03.005
physicianassistant.theclinics.com
2405-7991/16/$ – see front matter © 2016 Elsevier Inc. All rights reserved.

PATIENT CASE 1

It was Natalie's first day back to work on the inpatient oncology service after several days off. She joined her co-PAs, Kara and Joe, in the team office before rounds. She was assigned the care of 6 patients, 1 of whom was "complex," as Kara and Joe explained. After she received her patient assignments, Natalie made her way to the seventh floor to interview and examine this complex patient, who was known as "Dr H."

On chart review, Natalie learned that Dr H was an elderly man who had presented on hospital admission to the medical oncology ward 2 nights prior due to complaints of uncontrolled pain. His diagnosis was metastatic lung cancer, which had been diagnosed 2 years prior. Multiple organ systems were involved, including metastasis to the bones, liver, and kidneys. He had exhausted all conventional treatment options, and in fact he was still quite deconditioned from his most recent chemotherapy. He was being considered for a clinical trial, if his performance status were to improve.

Natalie recognized the patient as a well-known physician within the wider hospital system. Dr H lived with his wife, who was his health care proxy and caregiver. Although culturally Eastern European, he spoke English fluently. He was very religious, and the team had alluded to the fact that his religious beliefs strongly influenced his treatment decisions and his approach to death.

Dr H had multiple prior hospital admissions, during which time he had self-advocated for aggressive treatment. He wanted "everything done" in an effort to improve physically so that he might receive therapy with the clinical trial drug. During his prior hospital admissions, he had remained active and assertive in his medical decision making, although his wife was always present and they functioned as a cohesive team. The patient proudly identified as a physician, and he appreciated being referred to as "Dr H" by those who cared for him.

Natalie noted that the patient had expressed his wishes for full code at the time of hospital admission 2 nights ago. The medical team deemed him to have decision-making capacity. What made the case more complex, however, was that the patient's clinical status had declined significantly over the past 24 hours. The day prior, his primary oncologist had delivered the news to Dr H that he was no longer a candidate for the clinical trial drug because of his worsening prognosis. The patient was understandably disappointed. It was not clear, however, why Dr H had decided at the end of yesterday's shift that he no longer wanted treatment of his pain symptoms.

Dr H's daytime nurse, Melissa, met Natalie at the nursing station. She confirmed that Dr H had refused pain mediation overnight and that morning. As Natalie entered Dr H's room, she noted that he was quietly groaning. His wife was at his bedside and kindly greeted Natalie. Dr H acknowledged her also, answered her questions, and allowed her to examine him. Natalie noted his labored respirations, rapid heart rate, and elevated blood pressure. After Natalie's offer of pain medication, Dr H refused, although he would not explain his reason for refusal. Thereafter, he seemed somewhat uninterested in having a conversation. His wife motioned to Natalie to meet her outside of the room.

Natalie and Sarah, the social worker, spoke at length with the wife of Dr H. She explained how disappointed Dr H was about his ineligibility to participate in the clinical trial. He also understood and accepted his physical decline and poor prognosis. He wanted to prepare himself properly for his death, and part of this process included accepting suffering. Mrs H explained that their religious beliefs required suffering as a necessary means to honorably enter the afterlife. This was the reason behind Dr H refusing pain medication. Natalie and Sarah thanked Mrs H for her insight into the patient's wishes, and she agreed to them returning later to discuss these details with Dr H.

The attending physician, Dr Conn, arrived to begin rounds. Natalie reported on Dr H's condition, on his physical examination findings, and on her discussion with Mrs H. Dr Conn immediately became agitated regarding Dr H's refusal of pain medication. He stated, "This is absurd! This man is a physician—he knows better! Natalie, it is your job to convince him to accept pain medication today!" Natalie cringed, because convincing Dr H to accept pain medication was the last thing she wanted to do.

Ethical Case Analysis

Case 1 is an example of the complex medical, emotional, and spiritual needs of a cancer patient. The medical team may approach this case independently or with the help of an ethics consultation service. The following 3-step approach for considering the ethical concerns of case 1 may be considered:

- What are the medical and social facts?
  In the case of Dr H, it is important to understand the basic medical facts of Dr H's diagnosis, including his prognosis. It is also important to identify the contributing social facts, including family and friend support. **Table 1** includes a summary of what is known.

Table 1
Case 1 medical and social facts

Past Medical History	Past Social History
Metastatic lung cancer diagnosed 2 y prior	Well-known physician within the wider hospital system
Multiple organ systems affected	Lives with wife, who is health care proxy and caregiver
Has exhausted all conventional treatment options, no longer being considered for clinical trial due to worsening prognosis	Culturally Eastern European, speaks English
The patient has uncontrolled pain related to his advanced, terminal cancer diagnosis.	Religious values contribute to his approach to death

- What are the ethical concerns?
  At least 2 concerns in the case of Dr H may be identified:
  ○ Is it ethical to honor the wishes of a patient (who has capacity for decision making) who refuses pain medications because of religious reasons, despite physical signs that he is suffering?
  ○ Is it ethical for Dr Conn to pressure Natalie into convincing the patient to accept pain medication when Dr H has refused this treatment?

- What decision would provide optimal care for the patient?
  To determine the best course of action for patient care, the medical and/or ethical team should evaluate the pertinent ethical concerns of the case. A discussion of the 2 major ethical concerns pertaining to case 1 follows.

Treatment Refusal

Myth: Patients who refuse recommended medical treatment are misinformed and merely require more information about their disease and treatment options in order for them to consent to the recommended therapy.

Truth: Any type of medical treatment requires informed consent by the patient or by the person designated to make decisions for the patient (eg, health care proxy). This case highlights a common clinical situation, known as *treatment refusal*. Dr H refuses to receive recommended pain medication to treat pain associated with metastatic lung cancer.

A patient may legally refuse recommended medical treatment, provided the patient has capacity (eg, cognitive ability to make informed decisions).[2] The ethics (eg, morality) of a patient's treatment refusal, however, may not be readily apparent to the clinical team. From an ethical standpoint, it is most important for the clinical team to understand the patient's values and the reasons behind the treatment refusal. Investigation into a patient's values requires communication with the patient and/or family and friends of the patient. The process of uncovering this information often requires time and mutual trust.

In Dr H's case, his refusal of treatment is not related to his lack of information, knowledge, or understanding. As a physician, he is well educated regarding his disease process and treatment options. As Natalie discovered while discussing with Dr H's wife, Dr H's spiritual values are the primary reason behind his refusal of pain medication. The ethical dilemma in this case is secondary to a conflict of values between the patient and medical team. Dr Conn's primary value is to alleviate pain and suffering for his patient. Dr H most values adhering to practices that comply with his religious beliefs. The ethical deliberation in this case involves finding a mutually agreed-on solution to the conflict of values between the patient and physician.

The medical and/or ethical team should use all available resources to help mediate a difficult case such as this. Although ethics is not the same as law, law and ethics can overlap and inform each other. In Dr H's case, understanding legal implications regarding treatment refusal is helpful. If a patient is deemed by a medical team to have capacity, then the medical team must uphold the patient's refusal of treatment, even when this may lead to death.[2] The medical team should understand, however, the terms of the patient's refusal in detail.[2] Legally, if a patient is deemed not to have capacity, a medical team may treat the patient without the patient's consent on the basis that is in the best interest of the patient.[2]

The medical and/or ethical team may also use hospital policies pertaining to certain clinical situations to assist in clinical case mediation. For instance, if the hospital has a policy on pain control, the PA should become familiar with that policy. The hospital in which Dr H was being treated had a hospital pain policy that allows the clinical team authority to treat an incapacitated patient with physical signs of pain with pain medication, even if family members refuse. The policy, however, did not address patient pain medication refusal based on religious beliefs.

When a patient refuses recommended medical treatment, it is also important to consider whether there are other contributing factors:

- Has informed consent for the medical treatment been explained completely and in understandable terms?[2,3]
- If the patient is non–English speaking, has the informed consent been performed in the presence of an interpreter?
- Does a patient have the mental capacity to understand the details of his/her medical condition and prognosis?[2]
- Are there complicating underlying psychiatric conditions, such as depression or anxiety, preventing a patient's understanding of the recommended therapy?[2]

Religious beliefs may often be given as the reason behind treatment refusal.[4] The ethical principle of autonomy (eg, self-rule) allows for a patient to make medical decisions or refuse treatment based on religious beliefs.[5] Given the sacred importance of religious beliefs, clinicians often aim to honor patient treatment refusal based on faith values.[5] Treatment refusal based on religious reasons, however, should not be honored if the decision places society at risk (eg, treatment of infectious disease).[5] Some ethicists argue that a patient is not refusing the treatment, as much as refusing the religious implications of the treatment.[6] In Dr H's case, he refused pain medication because he did not want to lose the hope of entering the afterlife without appropriate religious honor.

Moral Distress

Myth: Clinicians rarely encounter situations in which they are morally compromised.

Fact: When caring for medically complex patients, clinicians may be asked by patients or other interdisciplinary team members to perform deeds that they feel are morally compromising. This case highlights a situation of moral distress, in which Natalie feels morally at odds when Dr Conn requests her to convince Dr H to accept pain medication. She has learned that Dr H's refusal of pain medication is related to his strong religious beliefs, and Natalie wishes to honor Dr H's values. Situations of moral distress consist of either internal (personal) or external (institutional) constraints that prevent a clinician from acting in a manner that is consistent with his/her moral values.[7] In other words, the clinician knows the right thing to do but feels unable to do the right thing. Natalie feels powerless to act according to her own moral standards because she fears conflict between herself and her boss, Dr Conn.

Moral distress is a common experience for clinicians and typically occurs because of conflicts over who is in charge, cost constraints on patient care, or controversial end-of-life scenarios.[8,9] Clinicians who provide direct patient care and those who provide end-of-life care in the ICU are particularly prone to moral distress.[10] Over time, repeated episodes of moral distress may lead to emotional distress, compassion fatigue, and clinician burnout.[9] When confronted with moral distress, it is important for an individual to take time to communicate with the interdisciplinary team regarding any team, unit, or system barriers to ethically appropriate patient care.[9] Although it requires moral courage to challenge the constraints to ethical patient care, it may be important for a clinician to do so.

PATIENT CASE 2

Leah was completing her day in oncology clinic and received a page from the inpatient ICU oncology team regarding her patient, George. Before returning the page, Leah reviewed his case. George was a 23-year-old man, found to have HIV at the time of his Hodgkin lymphoma diagnosis 2 years ago. As his clinic PA, Leah had followed George throughout his treatment of Hodgkin lymphoma. She had last evaluated him in clinic 6 months prior when George celebrated a complete remission confirmed by his 2-year post-treatment PET scan. Despite his intermittent noncompliance with antiretroviral medications, Leah thought that George would adhere to medication compliance after her counseling in clinic that day. She had emphasized how important taking his HIV medications was to help his immune system, and she reminded him that taking these medications would assist in continued lymphoma remission.

George had a complex social history. He lived with his mother and siblings, with whom he was very close. George's father was mostly absent, apart from intermittent visits at important holidays. His mother and father were technically still married; however, they lived separately and were not in close communication. George worked long hours at a warehouse to help provide financial support to his mother, siblings, and his sister's infant child. George had never been willing to assign a health care proxy, mostly because he could not decide between appointing his mother or father. George was concerned that his father might cease communication if he appointed his mother as his health care proxy.

When Leah reached the hospital team by phone, she learned that George's blood work on admission 1 week prior demonstrated a very low CD4 count and significant elevation of HIV viral load, indicating that George had not been compliant with his HIV medications. Unfortunately, George had developed a rapidly growing supraclavicular lymph node, which prompted his emergency department visit. Within several minutes of arriving to the emergency department, George developed respiratory distress due to external lymph node compression of his airway. The emergency room team had attempted intubation, but they had been unsuccessful due to extensive compromise of the airway. The ICU team had been contacted to assist, and ultimately, an emergent tracheostomy was placed. George was now being supported on a ventilator.

Over the past week, George had required placement of a percutaneous endoscopic gastrostomy tube for nutritional purposes. He had been sluggish to recover his neurologic status after tracheostomy placement, but his family remained hopeful. The case was further complicated by the fact that George had suffered a brain aneurysmal bleed the night prior, causing further deterioration in his neurologic status. Two separate neurologists had evaluated him, and he was determined to have an extensive brain hemorrhage. The ICU team had presented the option of either hospice care or a high-risk surgery. The surgery would require George to remain on a ventilator the rest of his life. At best, he would be awake and alert, although he would never live independently again and never regain full cognitive status. At worst, the surgery would leave George in a persistent vegetative state. Both his mother and father were at his bedside, but they had differing wishes for George. His mother stated that George had once told her that he would never want to live in this state. He had previously expressed his wishes to remain active, provide for his family, and to live an independent life. George's father asserted, however, that all measures should be taken to keep George alive. He wanted "everything done" and was still hoping that his son would recover after the risky surgery. The team was uncertain how to proceed regarding the surgery, given the parental disagreement.

The inpatient ICU team was seeking Leah's assistance because of her extensive knowledge of the patient. The ethics team had been called, and they were requesting that Leah be present at an upcoming family meeting, where the team was planning to have further discussion about medical decisions for George.

The Physician Assistant and Bioethics

The PA who cares for oncology patients has a unique role in the function of the interdisciplinary care team. As a knowledgeable clinician and because of the extent of time spent with a patient, the PA becomes familiar with details regarding the patient's medical case and social details. The PA may have an integral role in explaining complex medical information to the patient and family. For these reasons, the PA often becomes involved in advocating for the patient's values and may act as a mediator between the patient and other medical team members. The PA role is also unique because of the supervisory role of the attending physician. The American Academy of Physician Assistants (AAPA) "Guidelines for Ethical Conduct for the Physician Assistant Profession" encourages PAs to conduct themselves in the upmost legal and moral fashion. The AAPA includes 4 principles, introduced by Beauchamp and Childress, as guidelines for a PA's ethical conduct.[11]

Principle-Based Ethics

A common method used by medical/ethics teams to deliberate ethical concerns is the principle-based ethics model. Beauchamp and Childress founded this model, proposing that 4 main principles should govern the ethical decision making in the care of patients.[12] The 4 principles are as follows:

- Autonomy: "self rule"[12]
- Beneficence: "do good"[12]
- Nonmaleficence: "do no harm"[12]
- Justice: "fairness, equal allocation of resources"[12]

When considering case 2, the 4 principles may be helpful in determining the best care for George. Because George has lost his autonomy and no longer has capacity for his own decision making, family members must decide for him.[13] How might a decision be made for George that is beneficent (eg, in his best interest), and how might maleficence (eg, doing harm) be avoided? How should the ethics team determine which family member might best decide for George?

Surrogate Decision Making

Myth: If a patient does not have capacity for decision making, the medical team may make decisions for the patient, as long as it is in the best interest of the patient.

Fact: In cases of a patients too ill to make their own medical decisions, an appointed individual (eg, surrogate) should do so.[3] Ideally, a patient should preemptively appoint a friend or family member as a surrogate, in a legal document, such as a health care proxy document or in an advance directive.[3] In many emergent cases, however, a patient has not officially named a person to act on his/her behalf.[3] It is, therefore, the task of the medical team and/or ethics committee to determine which family member or friend will act on behalf of the patient and according to the patient's values.[3,14]

Grief and adjustment to a patient's serious medical condition may cause a surrogate to have difficulty making decisions for the patient.[14] In these cases, the medical team may offer assistance to the surrogate by recommending how decisions should be made.[3]

- The surrogate may make a treatment decision for the patient based on known preferences that the patient indicated in previous conversations.[3] This is known as *substituted judgment.*
- If a patient's preference for treatment is not known, the surrogate may make a treatment decision for the patient based on the best understanding of values and beliefs of the patient.[3] This is known as *best interest judgment.*

There are rare cases when an appointed surrogate makes a decision contrary to the best interest of the patient. If this occurs, the medical team is required to take measures to appoint a different family member or friend who will act in the best interest of the patient.[3] This process requires working together with the ethics committee and through court proceedings.[3]

In case 2, George's parents are still legally married, placing them in equal standing for surrogate decision making. The team might take into consideration, however, that George had previously discussed with his mother his preferences, including that he wanted to live a life that was functional and active, with the ability to earn finances to support his family. Given that George lives with his mother and she seems to know his preferences first hand, the team may decide that George's mother would most accurately act in his best interest. Cases such as this are complex, however, and sometimes require legal deliberation if a unified parental decision cannot be made. The goal of ethical deliberation in this case is to uncover the best interest for George and to determine how the team and family might best support his wishes. Leah and the other members of the team are an important contribution to the conversation regarding George's life values.

PATIENT CASE 3

Alison joined late afternoon rounds with the rest of the medical care team. As the patient's PA, she had many updates to provide after her care of Lila, a 9-month-old infant admitted with complications related to a rare form of leukemia. The infant was gravely ill and suffering from infectious complications due to a low white blood cell count. The recent chemotherapy regimen had only improved her blood counts transiently, and she now had neutropenia and fever. Multiple intravenous antibiotics were being administered for treatment of sepsis. She also had thrombocytopenia and was requiring frequent platelet transfusions.

Her loving parents were at her bedside 24 hours per day, advocating for her life and ongoing therapy. This was not the first time Lila's parents had been confronted with serious illness in their family. Two of their other children had been diagnosed with the same form of leukemia for which Lila was being treated. After multiple therapies, including a bone marrow transplant for one child, both children died. Lila's pediatric oncologist, Dr Caise, had communicated her poor prognosis to Lila's parents 4 days ago. He anticipated Lila's lifespan as days to weeks. He recommended transitioning to palliative care to keep her as comfortable as possible.

Lila's parents were not ready to stop treatment, and, therefore, they began investigating other treatment options. They discovered a recently available clinical trial, which would then need to be followed by a sibling-donor bone marrow transplant. The statistics for survival after this therapy were slim, estimated at no more than 10%. Without this therapy, however, Lila would certainly not survive. Lila had a 4-year-old sister, Katie, whom the parents volunteered as the bone marrow transplant donor.

As her colleagues gathered for rounds, Alison updated the team on the parents' wishes for the clinical trial therapy, followed by the sibling-donor bone marrow transplant. The team unanimously expressed their concerns that this therapy would be nonbeneficial for Lila. They were also concerned about the risks to Lila's sister, Katie, as the bone marrow donor. Dr Caise agreed with the team. He did not believe that Lila would survive the clinical trial therapy, and, given her current condition, he believed Lila might even die in the next few days.

Dr Caise and Alison met with Lila's parents to communicate his opinion that the clinical trial therapy would be nonbeneficial for Lila. Dr Caise also reiterated his concern for the Lila's guarded condition. The parents were very disappointed, and the next day, they began investigating the possibility of having Lila transferred to another institution where staff was willing to begin administering the clinical trial therapy. Lila was deemed too ill and unstable, however, to travel to another facility. The parents requested another meeting with Dr Caise, where they communicated their unwillingness to accept palliative care. They asked that Dr Caise and the team reconsider their wishes for the clinical trial therapy. They wanted "everything done." Dr Caise was at a standstill, so he requested an ethics consult to help assist with the care of Lila.

Pediatric Medical Care and Research in Children

Case 3 involves ethical concerns surrounding the medical and oncologic care of a child. Given a child's lack of autonomy, medical decisions for children require oversight by parents or other legally appointed guardian(s). It is important to consider unique aspects pertaining to the care of children.

Parental Permission/Assent

Myth: Children may not offer their opinion regarding medical treatment or research participation.

Fact: As learned from case 1, adults with capacity may consent to or refuse medical treatment after weighing the benefits and burdens of such therapy. Children (eg, those who are not of legal adult age) may not legally provide informed consent for medical treatment or research.[15] Therefore, parents of children or appointed guardians provide parental permission for their child's medical care and research participation.[15] The exception to this rule includes children who are considered emancipated minors.[15] Children who are "self-supporting and/or not living at home; married; pregnant or a parent; in the military; or declared to be 'emancipated by a court'" may provide informed consent for any medical treatment."[15]

In addition to parental permission, whenever possible and appropriate, children should be involved in decisions about their medical care.[16] A child's agreement to be involved in research, otherwise known as assent, is required unless the child is too young or too ill to participate.[15,17] Assent generally applies to children who are of intellectual age 7 years or older.[18] Elements of assent include the following:

- "Helping a patient achieve a developmentally appropriate awareness of the nature of his or her condition"[15]
- "Telling the patient what he or she can expect with tests and treatment(s)"[15]
- "Making a clinical assessment of the patient's understanding of the situation and the factors influencing how he or she is responding [to therapy]"[15]
- "Soliciting an expression of the patient's willingness to accept the proposed care…"[15]

Assent should be sought for all research treatments, particularly for participation in phase I clinical trials, when there may be no potential benefit to the patient.[15]

Clinicians may also face situations where parents refuse recommended treatment of a pediatric patient. It is not acceptable for a parent or guardian to refuse beneficial medical treatment of a child, even if religiously motivated.[5] Parental treatment refusal violates parental authority.[5] Parental responsibility includes protecting their children and assisting them to actualize their own autonomy.[5] If a medical team believes the parents are acting in a manner that places the safety of the child at risk, the medical team is permitted to assume decision making and act in the best interest of the child.[5]

Nonbeneficial Therapy

Myth: There are few requests for nonbeneficial therapy, especially in the care of pediatric patients.

Fact: Nonbeneficial treatment is treatment that is considered excessive, unsuccessful, or ineffective.[5] Nonbeneficial therapy has previously been referred to as "futile" therapy, although this term is not encouraged in the ethical literature because of its confusing definition.[19] Competent adult patients and parents of young children make medical decisions based on personal values and beliefs. Medical treatment requests are based on "what makes life meaningful and what burdens are acceptable."[16]

In the pediatric realm, clinicians and parents often disagree regarding the ability of a child to recover from a serious illness.[16] Parents are obligated, legally and ethically, to protect a child from harm and to advocate for his/her well-being.[16] In an effort to protect a child, however, a parent may be unable to realize that the child is dying.[16] In the case of Lila, her parents continue to hope for improvement from a rare leukemia, which has also claimed the lives of her 2 siblings. Despite being told that Lila's prognosis is poor, her parents continue to hope for reversal of her condition. Lila's parents advocate for additional cancer therapy that is projected to be ineffective by the medical team. The parents and the medical team hold differing opinions about the benefits and burdens of the novel therapy. Dr Caise considers the clinical trial therapy nonbeneficial, whereas Lila's parents consider the therapy their only hope for Lila's survival. Conflict arises because of differing values and goals.

In rare cases, nonbeneficial therapy is administered to pediatric patients even when the medical team is doubtful that it will be successful. In an effort to demonstrate to the parents that all efforts have been made to help the child, the medical team sometimes initiates/extends therapy they project will be ineffective. This includes cases of nonbeneficial cardiopulmonary resuscitation.[20] The practice of administering nonbeneficial care in children is controversial and is rarely applied in adults.

Bioethics Mediation

It is important for a medical team to recognize when a conflict of values/goals interferes with patient care. In order to deliberate a case in which the medical team and parents of the patient disagree on treatment, it is important to garner the support of the hospital ethics consultation team. In cases such as Lila's, the ethics consultation team will likely consider using a model known as *bioethics mediation*. Bioethics mediation is a concept developed by the bioethicist, Dubler and Liebman.[21] Bioethics mediation is a process that helps ethics consultants reach "principled resolutions" to complex conflicts.[21] Components of bioethics mediation and examples of how the components pertain to case 3 are listed in **Table 2**.

Table 2 Bioethics mediation steps for case 3	
Bioethics Mediation Components	**Case 3**
"Identify the parties to the conflict."[21]	Dr Caise, the medical team, and Lila's parents
"Minimize disparities of power, knowledge, skill, and experience" that contribute to the conflict.[21]	Take time to hear the facts of the case from all involved parties.
"Help the parties define their interests."[21]	Identify the values of Dr Caise/medical team (keeping the patient comfortable) and Lila's parents (extending Lila's life).
"Help maximize options for a resolution of the conflict."[21]	Present options for the care of Lila. Consider proposing a 3-day observation of Lila's condition and then meet again to discuss her care.
"Search for common ground or areas of consensus."[21]	Spend time discussing Lila's prognosis and investigate how the loss of Lila's siblings is contributing to the parents' current treatment requests.
"Ensure that the consensus can be justified as a principled resolution, compatible with the principles of bioethics and the legal rights of patient and families."[21]	Emphasize the common goal of care for Lila. Emphasize a care plan that will be in her best interest (beneficent) and without harm (nonmaleficent). Consider discussion of the fair use of resources (justice) as a means to explaining why the parents should carefully consider their request for the clinical trial therapy.

In patient case 3, bioethics mediation should include a discussion with all parties involved in the conflict. Additional team members may attend for clinician or family support, including social work and chaplaincy. In the case of Lila, a detailed discussion of Lila's prognosis should occur. The medical team may consider focusing on helping the parents adjust to the severity of the patient's illness. If Lila's parents are able to come to terms with her poor prognosis, they may acknowledge that she is a poor candidate for further cancer therapy. It is also helpful for the medical team to emphasize what is currently being done to help Lila because this will demonstrate to Lila's parents the shared goal of "doing good" for the patient. It may also be helpful to discuss the deaths of Lila's siblings and how those deaths affected the family. Discussing the loss of Lila's siblings may also help the medical team understand Lila's parents' current request for the novel clinical trial therapy. It also is important to discuss the potential risks of the clinical trial therapy and explain why the therapy is not in the best interest of Lila.

Hopefully these ethical discussions with Dr Caise, the medical team, Lila's parents, and the ethics consultation service may help both sides determine an agreeable plan for Lila's care. If conflict persists, it is sometimes helpful to propose meeting again in 1 to 3 days to reassess a patient's condition. For example, if the group meets again in 3 days and Lila continues to require antibiotics and transfusions, this may provide evidence that the patient is very ill and not a candidate for further cancer treatment. Placing time parameters on decision making and frequently reassessing a patient's clinical status are often helpful in coming to a mutually agreed-on decision for patient care. Communication between the involved parties is the best method for mediating conflict pertaining to values and goals.

SUMMARY/DISCUSSION

These 3 cases represent common ethical dilemmas encountered in the care of oncology patients. It is important for PAs to be aware of their unique role within the interdisciplinary team and how to navigate clinical ethical dilemmas. The ethical issues and methods for ethical deliberation discussed in this article are presented with the aim of helping PAs provide optimal care for cancer patients.

REFERENCES

1. Purtilo R, Doherty R. Ethical dimensions in the health professions. 5th edition. St Louis (MO): Elsevier; 2011.
2. Larner E, Carter L. The issue of consent in medical practice. Br J Haematol 2016; 172(2):300–4.
3. Terry P. Informed consent in clinical medicine. Chest 2007;131(2):563–8.
4. Burton LA, Bosek MS. When religion may be an ethical issue. J Relig Health 2000; 39(2):97–106.
5. Niebroj LT. The influence of religious beliefs on health care: between medical futility and refusal of treatment. J Physiol Pharmacol 2006;57(4):241–9.
6. Curlin FA, Roach CJ, Gorawara-Bhat R, et al. When patients choose faith over medicine: physician perspectives on religiously related conflict in the medical encounter. Arch Intern Med 2005;165(1):88–91.
7. Epstein EG, Hamric AB. Moral distress, moral residue, and the crescendo effect. J Clin Ethics 2009;20(4):330–42.
8. Crippen D. Moral distress in medicine: powerlessness by any other name. J Crit Care 2016;31(1):271–2.

9. Whitehead PB, Herbertson RK, Hamric AB, et al. Moral distress among health-care professionals: report of an institution-wide survey. J Nurs Scholarsh 2015; 47(2):117–25.

10. Hamric AB, Blackhall LJ. Nurse-physician perspectives on the care of dying patients in intensive care units: collaboration, moral distress, and ethical climate. Crit Care Med 2007;35(2):422–9.

11. Guidelines for ethical conduct for the physician assistant profession. Adopted 2000. Amended 2004, 2006, 2007, 2008. Reaffirmed 2013. The American Academy of Physician Assistants. Available at: https://www.aapa.org/WorkArea/DownloadAsset.aspx?id=815. Accessed January 23, 2016.

12. Beauchamp T, Childress J. Principles of biomedical ethics. 7th edition. Oxford (England): Oxford University Press; 2013.

13. Sulmasy DP, Terry PB, Weisman CS, et al. The accuracy of substituted judgments in patients with terminal diagnoses. Ann Intern Med 1998;128(8):621–9.

14. Scheunemann LP, Arnold RM, White DB. The facilitated values history: helping surrogates make authentic decisions for incapacitated patients with advanced illness. Am J Respir Crit Care Med 2012;186(6):480–6.

15. Informed consent, parental permission, and assent in pediatric practice.Committee on Bioethics, American Academy of Pediatrics. Pediatrics 1995;95(2):314–7.

16. Rushton CH. Ethics and palliative care in pediatrics. Am J Nurs 2004;104(4): 54–63.

17. Fleischman AR, Collogan LK. Research with children. In: Emanuel EJ, Grady C, Crouch RA, et al, editors. The oxford textbook of clinical research ethics. New York: Oxford University Press; 2008. p. 446–60.

18. Guidelines for the ethical conduct of studies to evaluate drugs in pediatric populations. Committee on drugs, American Academy of Pediatrics. Pediatrics 1995;95(2):286–94.

19. Troug RD, Brett AS, Frader J. Sounding board: the problem with futility. N Engl J Med 1992;326(23):1560–4.

20. Troug RD. Is it always wrong to perform futile CPR? N Engl J Med 2010;362(6): 477–9.

21. Dubler N, Liebman C. Bioethics mediation: a guide to shaping shared solutions. Special student edition. Nashville (TN): Vanderbilt University Press; 2011.

Printed and bound by CPI Group (UK) Ltd, Croydon, CR0 4YY

03/10/2024

01040391-0016